Math Competition Books S

Problem Solving Using the Rearrangement Inequality

Yongcheng Chen, Ph.D.

http://www.mymathcounts.com/index.php

Math Competition Books Series – The rearrangement inequality is a powerful problem-solving tool. For example, many fundamental inequalities, such as the AM-GM inequality, the Cauchy inequality, and the Chebyshev's inequality, can be generated from the rearrangement inequality.

This book shows how you can use the rearrangement inequality to solve a variety of problems.

The book can be used by students preparing for math competitions such as Mathcounts, AMC 10/12, AIME (American Invitational Mathematics Examination), and USAJMO/USAMO.

ISBN 9781470130350
BISAC: Education / Teaching Methods & Materials / Mathematics

Please contact mymathcounts@gmail.com for suggestions, corrections, or clarifications.

Table of Contents

This page is intentionally left blank.

Chapter 1. The Rearrangement Inequality Theorems

1. Introduction

Rearrangement Inequality is an interesting and powerful theorem which enables us to see the validity of many inequalities by inspection [1]. You can apply it in most unexpected circumstances. Coaches in the Math Olympiad training field call the rearrangement inequality "a wonderful inequality" and "one really useful inequality" [2], [3], [4].

In practice, Rearrangement inequality is strong. Many fundamental inequalities, e.g. the AM-GM inequality, the Cauchy inequality, and the Chebyshev's inequality, can be generated from the Rearrangement Inequality. Actually, the Rearrangement Inequality has been a result of fundamental importance in mathematics and in practice.

For cyclic inequalities, Rearrangement inequality seems to be very effective. However, sometimes it's not easy to realize the use of Rearrangement inequality because it is hidden after the normal order of variables is changed into chaos [5].

Since this theorem is much underused, being aware of Rearrangement inequality in a problem requires a bit more intuitive ability than for other inequalities [5].

However, this book will show you that this inequality is easy to learn, easy to use and yet a powerful tool in solving inequality problems.

2. A Notation of Cross Multiplication

We introduce a notation for the scalar products in this book.

This kind of notation first was introduced by Gauss in 1795 with the shoelace formula (also known as Gauss's area formula) that is a well-known formula in mathematical competitions to determine the area of a polygon whose vertices are described by their rectangular coordinates in the plane.

Let us say that we have two sequences $\{x_1, x_2, x_3\}$ and $\{y_1, y_2, y_3\}$.

We find the vertical products and do the sum using the following figure:
$S_1 = x_1 \cdot y_1 + x_2 \cdot y_2 + x_3 \cdot y_3$.

$$\begin{array}{ccc} x_1 & x_2 & x_3 \\ \downarrow & \downarrow & \downarrow \\ y_1 & y_2 & y_3 \end{array}$$

or $\begin{bmatrix} x_1 & x_2 & x_3 \\ \\ y_1 & y_2 & y_3 \end{bmatrix} = x_1y_1 + x_2y_2 + x_3y_3$

We find the following cross products and do the sum:
$S_2 = = x_1 \cdot y_2 + x_2 \cdot y_3 + x_3 \cdot y_1$.

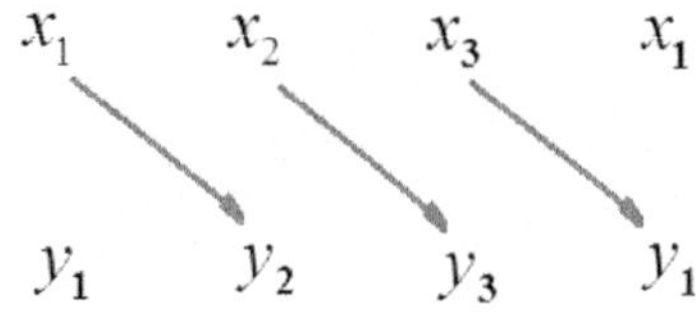

or $\begin{bmatrix} x_1 & x_2 & x_3 \\ \\ y_2 & y_3 & y_1 \end{bmatrix} = x_1y_2 + x_2y_3 + x_3y_1$

We find the following cross products and do the sum:
$S_3 = y_1 \cdot x_2 + y_2 \cdot x_3 + y_3 \cdot x_1$.

$$\begin{array}{cccc} x_1 & x_2 & x_3 & x_1 \\ \nearrow & \nearrow & \nearrow & \\ y_1 & y_2 & y_3 & y_1 \end{array}$$

or $\begin{bmatrix} x_1 & x_2 & x_3 \\ \\ y_3 & y_1 & y_2 \end{bmatrix} = x_1y_3 + x_2y_1 + x_3y_2$

We perform the following cross products and do the sum:
$S_4 = x_1y_3 + x_2y_2 + x_3y_1$

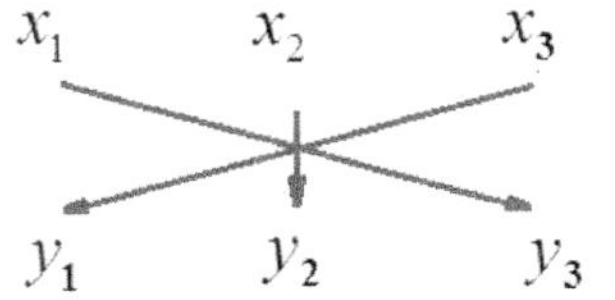

$x_1 \qquad x_2 \qquad x_3$

$y_1 \qquad y_2 \qquad y_3$

or $\begin{bmatrix} x_1 & x_2 & x_3 \\ & & \\ y_3 & y_2 & y_1 \end{bmatrix} = x_1y_3 + x_2y_2 + x_3y_1$

We perform the following cross products and do the sum:
$S_5 = x_1 \cdot y_1 + x_2 \cdot y_3 + x_3 \cdot y_2$.

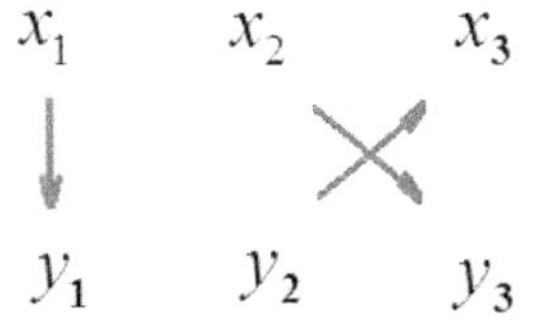

$x_1 \qquad x_2 \qquad x_3$

$y_1 \qquad y_2 \qquad y_3$

or $\begin{bmatrix} x_1 & x_2 & x_3 \\ & & \\ y_1 & y_3 & y_2 \end{bmatrix} = x_1y_1 + x_2y_3 + x_3y_2$

We perform the following cross products and do the sum:
$S_6 = x_1 \cdot y_2 + y_1 \cdot x_2 + x_3 \cdot y_3$.

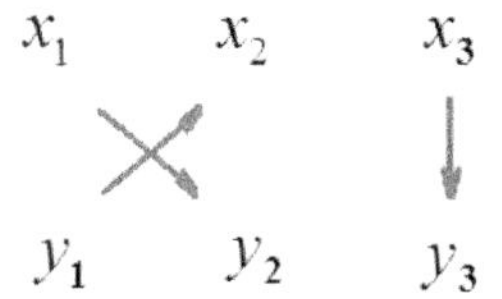

$x_1 \qquad x_2 \qquad x_3$

$y_1 \qquad y_2 \qquad y_3$

or $\begin{bmatrix} x_1 & x_2 & x_3 \\ & & \\ y_2 & y_1 & y_3 \end{bmatrix} = x_1y_2 + x_2y_1 + x_3y_3$

For the sequences $\{a, b, c, d\}$ and $\{a^2, b^2\ c^2, d^2\}$ with $0 \le a \le b \le c \le d$, we can have $4! = 24$ ways to express the sum of the products. Four of them are shown below.
We can have $S_1 = a^3 + b^3 + c^3 + d^3$.

$$\begin{array}{cccc} a & b & c & d \\ \downarrow & \downarrow & \downarrow & \downarrow \\ a^2 & b^2 & c^2 & d^2 \end{array}$$

or $\begin{bmatrix} a & b & c & d \\ a^2 & b^2 & c^2 & d^2 \end{bmatrix} = a^3 + b^3 + c^3 + d^3$

We have $S_2 = ab^2 + bc^2 + cd^2 + da^2$

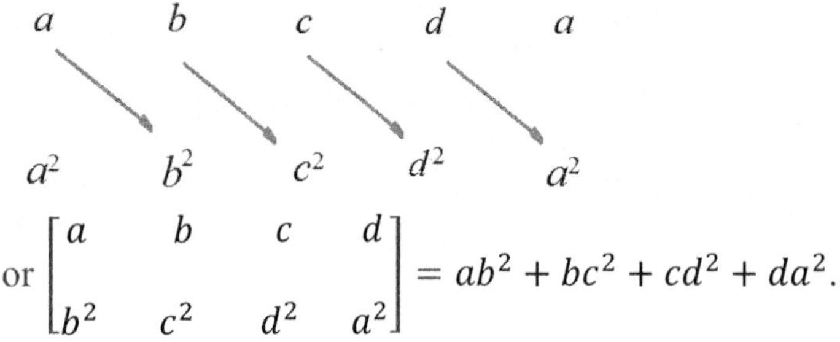

or $\begin{bmatrix} a & b & c & d \\ b^2 & c^2 & d^2 & a^2 \end{bmatrix} = ab^2 + bc^2 + cd^2 + da^2.$

We have $S_3 = ad^2 + ba^2 + cb^2 + dc^2$

$$\begin{array}{ccccc} a & b & c & d & a \\ \nearrow & \nearrow & \nearrow & \nearrow & \\ a^2 & b^2 & c^2 & d^2 & a^2 \end{array}$$

or $\begin{bmatrix} a & b & c & d \\ d^2 & a^2 & b^2 & c^2 \end{bmatrix} = ad^2 + ba^2 + cb^2 + dc^2.$

We have $S_4 = ad^2 + bc^2 + cb^2 + da^2$

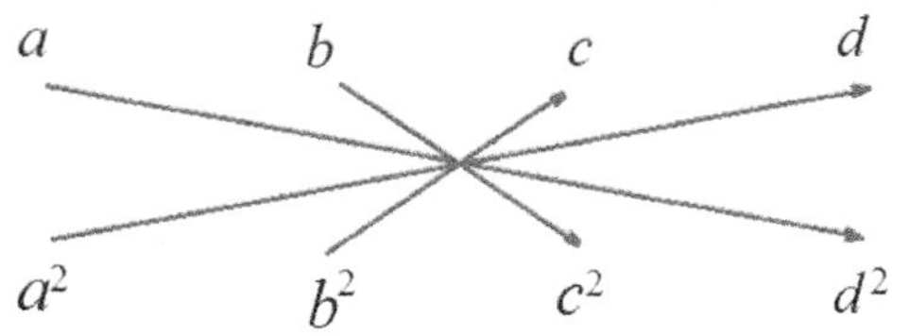

$a \quad b \quad c \quad d$

$a^2 \quad b^2 \quad c^2 \quad d^2$

or $\begin{bmatrix} a & b & c & d \\ d^2 & c^2 & b^2 & a^2 \end{bmatrix} = ad^2 + bc^2 + cb^2 + da^2.$

3. An Example of Rearrangement Inequality

Example 1. Three boxes contain \$10, \$100, and \$50 bills, respectively. You can take 2, 1, or 5 bills from each box. What is the smallest amount you can get?

Solution:
If we rearrange \$10, \$50, and \$100 in ascending order as a sequence $\{a_k\}$ $\{10, 50, 100\}$ and 1, 2, 5 in ascending order as well as another sequence $\{b_k\}$, (k is from 1 to 3), we have $3! = 6$ ways to express the sums of the products of a_k and b_k.

\$10 \$50 \$100
1 2 5

The greatest value is achieved when a_k and b_k are similarly ordered:

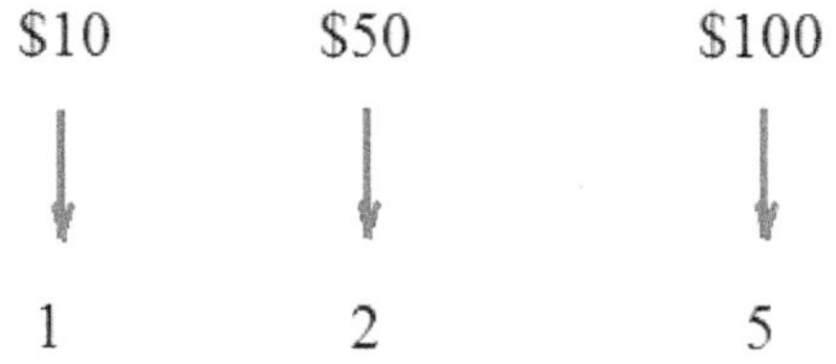

\$10 \$50 \$100

↓ ↓ ↓

1 2 5

The operation is done: $10 \times 1 + 50 \times 2 + 100 \times 5 = \$610$.

The smallest value is achieved when a_k and b_k are opposite ordered:

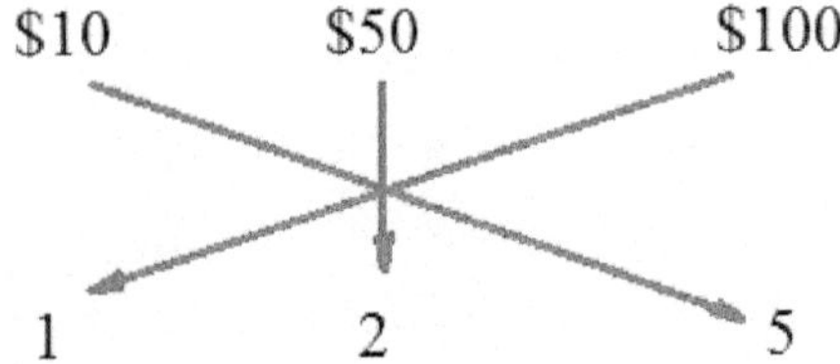

The operation is done: $10 \times 5 + 100 \times 1 + 50 \times 2 = \$250$.

The values between the greatest and the smallest are obtained when a_k and b_k are neither similarly nor opposite ordered (we have 4 cases):

(*a*) The operation is done: $10 \times 2 + 50 \times 5 + 100 \times 1 = \$370$.

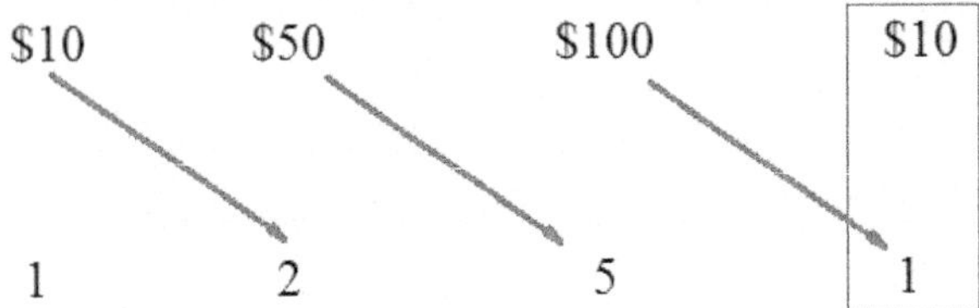

(*b*) The operation is done: $1 \times 50 + 2 \times 100 + 5 \times 10 = \$300$.

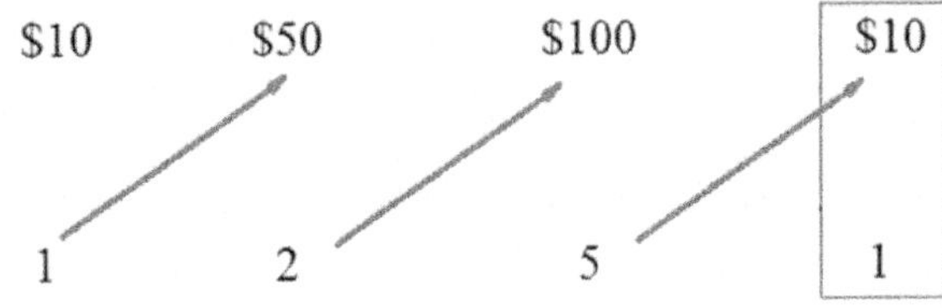

(*c*) The operation is done: $10 \times 1 + 50 \times 5 + 100 \times 2 = \$460$.

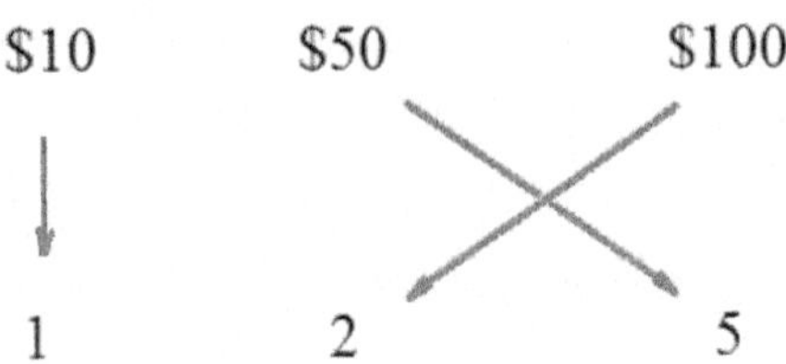

(*d*) The operation is done: $10 \times 2 + 50 \times 1 + 100 \times 5 = \$570$.

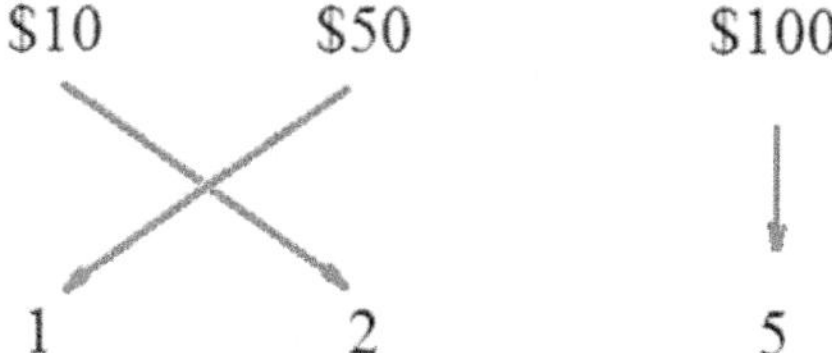

In order to pair \$100, sometimes we move the first column to the end.

It is clear that the maximum corresponds to similar ordering of $\{a_k\}$ and $\{b_k\}$,
$S = a_1b_1 + a_2b_2 + a_3b_3$
and the minimum corresponds to opposite ordering of $\{a_k\}$ and $\{b_k\}$.
$O = a_1b_3 + a_3\,b_1 + a_2b_2$

Between the maximum and the minimum, if a_k and b_k are neither similarly nor opposite ordered, we have P.

That is, we always have $S \geq P \geq O$ (1)

Hardy, Littlewood, and Polya [6] interpret the a_k as fixed distances along a rod and the b_k as weights to be suspended at these distances: To get the maximum moment with respect to an end of the rod hang the heaviest weights furthest from that end; to get the minimum moment hang the heaviest weights closest.

4. Rearrangement Inequality Theorems

4.1. Rearrangement Inequality Theorem I

For two real sequences $\{a_k\}$ and $\{b_k\}$, (k is from 1 to n, and n is a positive integer), we may rearrange the terms $\{a_k\}$ and $\{b_k\}$ in ascending order:

$a_1 \le a_2 \le a_3 \cdots \le a_n,$

$b_1 \le b_2 \le b_3 \cdots \le b_n,$

The maximum corresponds to similar ordering of $\{a_k\}$ and $\{b_k\}$,

$S = a_1b_1 + a_2b_2 + a_3b_3 + \cdots + a_nb_n$

and the minimum corresponds to opposite ordering of $\{a_k\}$ and $\{b_k\}$.

$O = a_nb_1 + a_{n-1}b_2 + a_{n-2}b_3 + \cdots + a_1b_n$

Between the maximum and the minimum, we have

$P = a_1b_1' + a_2b_2' + a_3b_3' + \cdots + a_nb_n'$

where $\{b_k'\}$ is any permutation of $\{b_k\}$.

That is, we have $S \ge P \ge O$

Proof:

(1) We prove $S \ge P$ first.

$a_1 \le a_2 \le a_3 \cdots \le a_n,$

$b_1 \le b_2 \le b_3 \cdots \le b_n,$

The maximum corresponds to similar ordering of $\{a_k\}$ and $\{b_k\}$,

$S = a_1b_1 + a_2b_2 + a_3b_3 + \cdots + a_nb_n$

$P = a_1b_1' + a_2b_2' + a_3b_3' + \cdots + a_nb_n'$

where $\{b_k'\}$ is any permutation of $\{b_k\}$.

Let a_n pair with b_n' ($b_n' \le b_n$), b_n pair with a_k ($k < n$)

Then $a_nb_n + a_kb_n' - a_kb_n - a_nb_n'$

$= (a_n - a_k)(b_n - b_n') \ge 0 \qquad \Rightarrow \qquad a_nb_n + a_kb_n' \ge a_kb_n + a_nb_n'$

Therefore, only when a_n pairs with b_n, P gets the greatest value.

Similarly, only when a_{n-1} pairs with b_{n-1}, a_{n-2} pairs with b_{n-2}, …., a_1 pairs with b_1, P gets the greatest value.

Thus $a_1b_1' + a_2b_2' + a_3b_3' + \cdots + a_nb_n' \le a_1b_1 + a_2b_2 + a_3b_3 + \cdots + a_nb_n$.
Equality holds if and only if $a_1 = a_2 = \ldots = a_n$ or $b_1 = b_2 = \ldots = b_n$.

(2) We prove $P \ge O$.
We have
$a_1 \le a_2 \le a_3 \cdots \le a_n$,
$-b_n \le -b_{n-1} \le b_{n-2} \le \ldots \le -b_2 \le -b_1$

Since $S \ge P$, we have
$a_1(-b_n) + a_2(-b_{n-1}) + a_3(-b_{n-2}) + \cdots + a_n(-b_1) \ge a_1(-b_1') + a_2(-b_2') + a_3(-b_3') + \cdots + a_n(-b_n')$
$\Rightarrow a_1b_n + a_2b_{n-1} + a_3b_{n-2} + \cdots + a_nb_1 \ge a_1b_1' + a_2b_2' + a_3b_3' + \cdots + a_nb_n'$

Equality holds if and only if $a_1 = a_2 = \ldots = a_n$ or $-b_n = -b_{n-1} = b_{n-2} = \ldots = -b_2 = -b_1$ $(b_1 = b_2 = \ldots = b_n)$.

Example 1. Show that $S \ge P \ge O$ for two sequences {2, 6, 7) and {3, 9, 12}.

Solution:
These two sequences are similarly ordered.
We see that
$S = 2 \cdot 3 + 6 \cdot 9 + 7 \cdot 12 = 144$.
$O = 2 \cdot 12 + 7 \cdot 3 + 6 \cdot 9 = 99$.
$P = 2 \cdot 9 + 6 \cdot 12 + 7 \cdot 3 = 111$.
$144 \ge 111 \ge 99$.
$S \ge P \ge O$.

Example 2. Show that $S \ge O$ when $n = 2$ for Rearrangement Inequality Theorem I.

Solution:
Method 1:

$a_1 \le a_2$ and $b_1 \le b_2$
Method 1:
$S = (a_1b_1 + a_2b_2)$
$O = a_1b_2 + a_2b_1$

$S - O = a_1b_1 + a_2b_2 - a_1b_2 - a_2b_1$
$= (a_2b_2 - a_1b_2) - (a_2b_1 - a_1b_1)$
$= b_2(a_2 - a_1) - b_1 (a_2 - a_1)$
$= (a_2 - a_1)(b_2 - b_1) \ge 0$

Method 2:
We have $(a_2 - a_1)(b_2 - b_1) \ge 0 \quad \Leftrightarrow \quad a_2b_2 - a_1b_2 - a_2b_1 + a_1b_1 \ge 0$
$\Leftrightarrow \quad (a_2b_2 + a_1b_1) - (a_1b_2 + a_2b_1) \ge 0.$
So $S \ge O.$

The equality holds only and only if $a_1 = a_2$ or $b_1 = b_2$.

Example 3. Show that $S \ge P \ge O$ when $n = 3$ for Rearrangement Inequality Theorem I.

Solution:
$a_1 \le a_2 \le a_3$
$b_1 \le b_2 \le b_3$
$S = a_1b_1 + a_2b_2 + a_3b_3$
$O = a_1b_3 + a_3b_1 + a_2b_2$
$P = a_1b_2 + a_2b_3 + a_3b_1$

$S - O = a_1b_1 + a_3b_3 - a_1b_3 - a_3b_1$
$= (a_3b_3 - a_3b_1) - (a_1b_3 - a_1b_1)$
$= a_3(b_3 - b_1) - a_1 (b_3 - b_1)$
$= (b_3 - b_1)(a_3 - a_1) \ge 0$

$P - O = a_1b_2 + a_2b_3 + a_3b_1 - a_1b_3 - a_3b_1 - a_2b_2$
$= (a_1b_2 - a_1b_3) + (a_2b_3 - a_2b_2)$
$= - a_1 (b_3 - b_2) + a_2 (b_3 - b_2)$
$= (b_3 - b_2)(a_2 - a_1) \ge 0$

$S - P = a_1b_1 + a_2b_2 + a_3b_3 - a_1b_2 - a_2b_3 - a_3b_1$
$= (a_1b_1 - a_3b_1) + (a_3b_3 - a_2b_3) + (a_2b_2 - a_1b_2)$
$= -b_1(a_3 - a_1) + b_3(a_3 - a_2) + b_2(a_2 - a_1)$

We know that $(a_3 - a_1) \geq (a_3 - a_2)$
So we have
$S - P = -b_1(a_3 - a_1) + b_3(a_3 - a_2) + b_2(a_2 - a_1)$
$\geq -b_1(a_3 - a_2) + b_3(a_3 - a_2) + b_2(a_2 - a_1)$
$= (a_3 - a_2)(-b_1 + b_3) + b_2(a_2 - a_1) \geq 0.$

Thus $S \geq P \geq O$.
The equality holds only and only if $a_1 = a_2 = a_3$ or $b_1 = b_2 = b_3$.

4.2. Rearrangement Inequality Theorem II

Let $a_1 \leq a_2 \leq \cdots \leq a_n$ and $b_1 \leq b_2 \leq \cdots \leq b_n$ be two increasing sequences of non-negative real numbers.
Among all possible products $(a_1 + b_{\sigma_1})(a_2 + b_{\sigma_2})(a_3 + b_{\sigma_3}) \cdots (a_n + b_{\sigma n})$
where σ_1 , σ_2 , $\cdots$ σ_n is a permutation of $(1, 2, 3, \ldots n)$.

$(a_1 + b_1)(a_2 + b_2) \cdots (a_n + b_n) \leq (a_1 + b_{\sigma_1})(a_2 + b_{\sigma_2}) \cdots (a_n + b_{\sigma n}) \leq (a_1 + b_n)(a_2 + b_{n-1})$
$\cdots (a_n + b_1)$.

Proof:
Take any random product $(a_1 + b_{\sigma_1})(a_2 + b_{\sigma_2}) \cdots (a_n + b_{\sigma n})$ which is not $(a_1 + b_1)(a_2 + b_2) \cdots (a_n + b_n)$.
There exits $i < j$ such that $b_{\sigma_i} > b_{\sigma_j}$.

If we exchange σ_i and σ_j, only two terms are changed. In that case, consider the two products
$(a_i + b_{\sigma_i})(a_j + b_{\sigma_j})$ and $(a_i + b_{\sigma_j})(a_j + b_{\sigma_i})$
$(a_i + b_{\sigma_i})(a_j + b_{\sigma_j}) - (a_i + b_{\sigma_j})(a_j + b_{\sigma_i}) = (a_i - a_j)(b_{\sigma_i} + b_{\sigma_j}) \geq 0.$

This mean exchanging σ_i and σ_j yields a larger or equal result.
In a similar manner we can prove that the product $(a_1 + b_n)(a_2 + b_{n-1})\cdots(a_n + b_1)$ is the maximum.

It follows that
$(a_1 + b_1)(a_2 + b_2)\cdots(a_n + b_n) \leq (a_1 + b_{\sigma_1})(a_2 + b_{\sigma_2})\cdots(a_n + b_{\sigma n}) \leq (a_1 + b_n)(a_2 + b_{n-1})$ $\cdots(a_n + b_1)$.

4.3. Generalization of Rearrangement Inequality Theorem

Another natural direction of generalizing the rearrangement inequality (I and II) is to consider the case in which there are more than two sequences of non-negative numbers. The theorems are given by Rearrangement Inequality Theorems III and IV. The proof of Theorem III and IV is essentially the same as that of Theorems I and II, and is therefore omitted[12][13].

4.3.1. Rearrangement Inequality Theorem III

Let $a_{k1} \leq a_{k2} \leq \cdots \leq a_{kn}$ $(k = 1, 2, \ldots m)$ be increasing sequences of non-negative real numbers and $b_1 \leq b_2 \leq \cdots \leq b_n$ be two increasing sequences of non-negative real numbers.

$a_{11} \leq a_{12} \leq a_{13} \cdots \leq a_{1n}$
$a_{21} \leq a_{22} \leq a_{23} \cdots \leq a_{2n}$
$\ldots \quad \ldots \quad \ldots$
$a_{m1} \leq a_{m2} \leq a_{m3} \cdots \leq a_{mn}$

If we take one number from each row and multiply them together and repeat the process until we finish for all the numbers, then we add all the products together. Among all the sums, the following one has the maximum value:
$S = a_{11}a_{21} \cdots a_{m1} + a_{12}a_{22} \cdots a_{m2} + \cdots + a_{1n}\, a_{2n} \cdots a_{mn}$.

Note: There is no equivalent of the *minimum* sum.

4.3.2 Rearrangement Inequality Theorem IV

Let $a_{k1} \le a_{k2} \le \cdots \le a_{kn}$ $(k = 1, 2, \ldots m)$ be increasing sequences of non-negative real numbers, and $b_1 \le b_2 \le \cdots \le b_n$ be two increasing sequences of non-negative real numbers.

$$
\begin{array}{l}
a_{11} \le a_{12} \le a_{13} \cdots \le a_{1n} \\
a_{21} \le a_{22} \le a_{23} \cdots \le a_{2n} \\
\ldots \quad \ldots \quad \ldots \\
a_{m1} \le a_{m2} \le a_{m3} \cdots \le a_{mn}
\end{array}
$$

If we take one number from each row and add them together and repeat the process until we finish for all the numbers, then we multiply these sum together. Among all the products, the following one has the minimum value:
$(a_{11} + a_{21} + \cdots + a_{m1})(a_{12} + a_{22} + \cdots + a_{m2}) \cdots (a_{1n} + a_{2n} + \cdots + a_{mn})$.

Chapter 2. Solving Problems Using Similarly Ordered Sequences

1. Commonly used similarly ordered sequences

Generally, the following pairs of sequences are similarly ordered:

a, b, c
a, b, c

a, b, c
$a^2, b^2\ c^2$

$a, \ b, \ c$
$a^n, b^n\ c^n$

a^n, b^n, c^n
a^m, b^m, c^m

$a, \ b, c, \ d$
$a^2, b^2\ c^2, d^2$

a, b, c, d
$a^3, b^3\ c^3, d^3$

a, b, c, d
$a^n, b^n\ c^n, d^n$

a, b, c
$\frac{1}{c}, \frac{1}{b}, \frac{1}{a}$

a, b, c
$\frac{1}{bc}, \frac{1}{ac}, \frac{1}{ab}$

$a, \quad b, \quad c$

$\frac{1}{b+c}, \frac{1}{a+c}, \frac{1}{a+b}$

$a^2, \quad b^2 \quad c^2$

$\frac{1}{b+c}, \frac{1}{a+c}, \frac{1}{a+b}$

$a^3, b^3\ c^3$

$\frac{1}{b+c}, \frac{1}{a+c}, \frac{1}{a+b}$

$\frac{a}{b}, \frac{b}{c}, \frac{c}{a}$

$\frac{a}{b}, \frac{b}{c}, \frac{c}{a}$

The above similarly sorted sequences can be generalized to three sequences.

$a, \ b, \ c$

$a, \ b, \ c$

$a, b, \ c$

$a, \quad b, \ c$

$a, \quad b, \ c$

$a^3, b^3\ c^3$

$a, \quad b, \ c$

$a^2, b^2\ c^2$

$a^2, b^2\ c^2$

Example 1. *a, b* are positive real numbers. Show that $a^2 + b^2 \geq 2ab$.

Solution:
We have the following two similarly ordered sequences:

a, b

a, b

By the rearrangement inequality, we have

$$\begin{matrix} a & b \\ \downarrow & \downarrow \\ a & b \end{matrix} \qquad \begin{matrix} a & & b \\ & \times & \\ a & & b \end{matrix}$$

or $\begin{bmatrix} a & b \\ a & b \end{bmatrix} \geq \begin{bmatrix} a & b \\ b & a \end{bmatrix}$

$a \cdot a + b \cdot b = a^2 + b^2 \geq a \cdot b + a \cdot b = 2ab.$
Equality of this inequality occurs if and only if $a = b$.

Example 2. Prove that $\frac{a}{\sqrt{b}} + \frac{b}{\sqrt{a}} \geq \sqrt{a} + \sqrt{b}$ for positive values of a and b.

Proof:
Method 1:
If $a \leq b$, then $\frac{1}{\sqrt{b}} \leq \frac{1}{\sqrt{a}}$; If $a \geq b$, then $\frac{1}{\sqrt{b}} \geq \frac{1}{\sqrt{a}}$. So we have the following two similarly ordered sequences:

a, b

$\frac{1}{\sqrt{b}}, \frac{1}{\sqrt{a}}$

By the rearrangement inequality, we have

$$\begin{matrix} a & b \\ \downarrow & \downarrow \\ \frac{1}{\sqrt{b}} & \frac{1}{\sqrt{a}} \end{matrix} \qquad \begin{matrix} a & & b \\ & \times & \\ \frac{1}{\sqrt{b}} & & \frac{1}{\sqrt{a}} \end{matrix}$$

or $\begin{bmatrix} \sqrt{a} & \sqrt{b} \\ \frac{1}{\sqrt{b}} & \frac{1}{\sqrt{a}} \end{bmatrix} \geq \begin{bmatrix} \sqrt{a} & \sqrt{b} \\ \frac{1}{\sqrt{a}} & \frac{1}{\sqrt{b}} \end{bmatrix}$.

$\frac{a}{\sqrt{b}} + \frac{b}{\sqrt{a}} \geq a \cdot \frac{1}{\sqrt{a}} + b \cdot \frac{1}{\sqrt{b}} = \sqrt{a} + \sqrt{b}$.
The equality holds if and only if $a = b$.

Method 2:
We know that for positive values of a and b,

$a + b \geq 2\sqrt{ab}$ (1)

Dividing both sides of (1) by $\sqrt{b}$:

$\frac{a}{\sqrt{b}} + \sqrt{b} \geq 2\sqrt{a}$ (2)

Dividing both sides of (1) by $\sqrt{a}$:

$\sqrt{a} + \frac{b}{\sqrt{a}} \geq 2\sqrt{b}$ (3)

(2) + (3):

$\frac{a}{\sqrt{b}} + \sqrt{b} + \sqrt{a} + \frac{b}{\sqrt{a}} \geq 2\sqrt{a} + 2\sqrt{b} \Rightarrow \frac{a}{\sqrt{b}} + \frac{b}{\sqrt{a}} \geq \sqrt{a} + \sqrt{b}$.

The equality holds if and only if $a = b$.

Example 3. Show that $a^2 + b^2 + c^2 \geq ab + bc + ca$. a, b, c are positive.

Proof:
For the two similarly ordered sequences
a, b, c
a, b, c

by the rearrangement inequality, we have

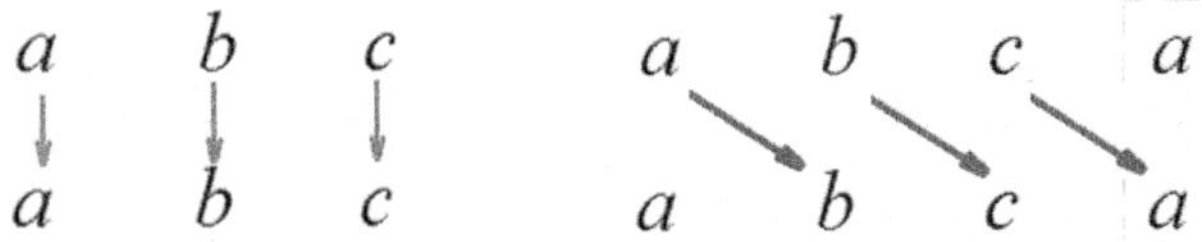

We have $a^2 + b^2 + c^2 \geq ab + bc + ca$.

Example 4. Show that if both *a* and *b* are positive real numbers, then $a^3 + b^3 \geq a^2b + ab^2$.

Solution:

We know that the following two similarly ordered sequences:

a, b

a^2, b^2

By the rearrangement inequality, we have

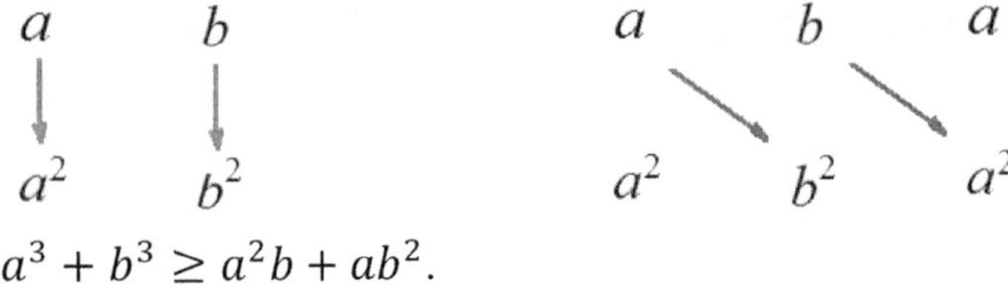

$a^3 + b^3 \geq a^2b + ab^2$.

Example 5. If $a, b, c \geq 0$, show $a^3 + b^3 + c^3 \geq 3abc$.

Solution:

For the following similarly ordered sequences,

a, b, c

a, b, c

a, b, c

By the rearrangement inequality, we have

$a \quad b \quad c \qquad a \quad b \quad c \quad a \quad b$

$a \quad b \quad c \qquad a \quad b \quad c \quad a \quad b$

$a \quad b \quad c \qquad a \quad b \quad c \quad a \quad b$

$a^3 + b^3 + c^3 \geq abc + abc + abc = 3abc$.

Example 6. If a, b, $c \geq 0$, show that $a^5 + b^5 + c^5 \geq abc\,(a^2 + b^2 + c^2)$.

Proof:

For the following similarly ordered sequences,

$a, \ b, \ c$

$a, \ b, \ c$

$a^3, b^3\ c^3$

By the rearrangement inequality, we have

$$\begin{array}{ccc} a & b & c \\ \downarrow & \downarrow & \downarrow \\ a & b & c \\ \downarrow & \downarrow & \downarrow \\ a^3 & b^3 & c^3 \end{array} \qquad \begin{array}{ccccc} a & b & c & a & b \\ & \searrow & \searrow & \searrow & \\ a & b & c & a & b \\ & \searrow & \searrow & \searrow & \\ a^3 & b^3 & c^3 & a^3 & b^3 \end{array}$$

$a^5 + b^5 + c^5 \geq abc^3 + bca^3 + cab^3 \geq abc(a^2 + b^2 + c^2)$.

Example 7. Show that if both a, b and c are positive numbers, then $(a + b)(b + c)(c + a) \geq 8abc$

Solution:

Method 1:

We have the following two similarly ordered sequences:

$\sqrt{a}\,, \sqrt{b}$

$\sqrt{a}\,, \sqrt{b}$

By the rearrangement inequality, we have

$$\begin{array}{cc} \sqrt{a} & \sqrt{b} \\ \downarrow & \downarrow \\ \sqrt{a} & \sqrt{b} \end{array} \qquad \begin{array}{ccc} \sqrt{a} & & \sqrt{b} \\ & \times & \\ \sqrt{a} & & \sqrt{b} \end{array}$$

$$\sqrt{a}\cdot\sqrt{a} + \sqrt{b}\cdot\sqrt{b} = a + b \geq \sqrt{a}\cdot\sqrt{b} + \sqrt{a}\cdot\sqrt{b} = 2\sqrt{ab} \qquad (1)$$

We can have the following two similarly ordered sequences:

$\sqrt{b}\,, \sqrt{c}$

$\sqrt{b}\,, \sqrt{c}$

By the rearrangement inequality, we have

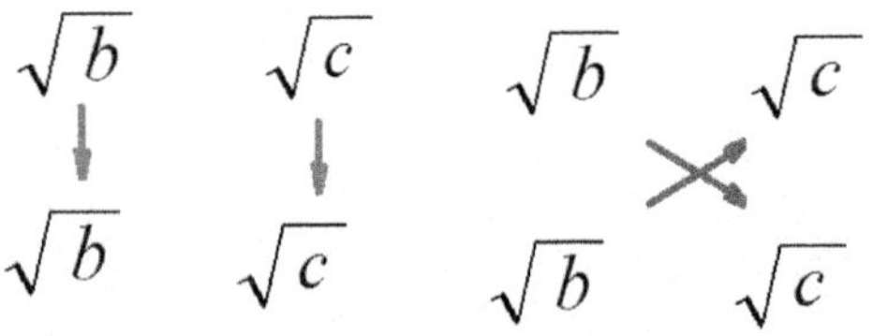

$$\begin{array}{cccc} \sqrt{b} & \sqrt{c} & \sqrt{b} & \sqrt{c} \\ \downarrow & \downarrow & \times & \\ \sqrt{b} & \sqrt{c} & \sqrt{b} & \sqrt{c} \end{array}$$

$\sqrt{b}\cdot\sqrt{b}+\sqrt{c}\cdot\sqrt{c}=b+c\ge\sqrt{b}\cdot\sqrt{b}+\sqrt{c}\cdot\sqrt{c}=2\sqrt{bc}$ (2)

We can have the following two similarly ordered sequences:

$\sqrt{c}\,,\sqrt{a}$

$\sqrt{c}\,,\sqrt{a}$

By the rearrangement inequality, we have

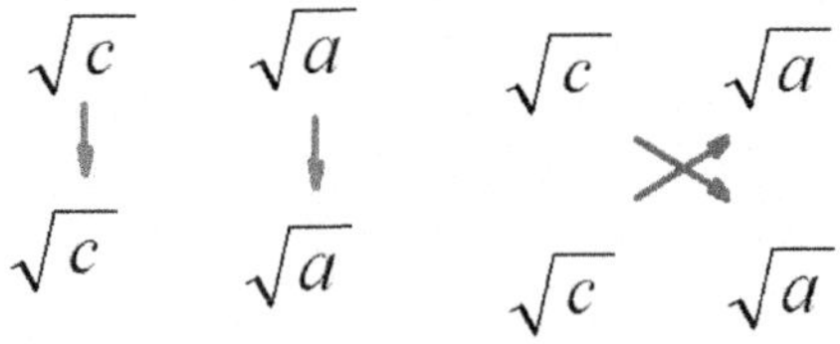

$$\begin{array}{cccc} \sqrt{c} & \sqrt{a} & \sqrt{c} & \sqrt{a} \\ \downarrow & \downarrow & \times & \\ \sqrt{c} & \sqrt{a} & \sqrt{c} & \sqrt{a} \end{array}$$

$\sqrt{c}\cdot\sqrt{c}+\sqrt{a}\cdot\sqrt{a}=c+a\ge\sqrt{c}\cdot\sqrt{a}+\sqrt{c}\cdot\sqrt{a}=2\sqrt{ca}$ (3)

$(1)\times(2)\times(3)$:

$(a+b)(b+c)(c+a)\ge\left(2\sqrt{ab}\right)\left(2\sqrt{bc}\right)\left(2\sqrt{ca}\right)=8abc$

Method 2:

We have the following two similarly ordered sequences:

$a, b, c.$

$a, b, c.$

By the Rearrangement Inequality Theorem II, we have

$(a+a)(b+b)(c+c)\le(a+b)(b+c)(c+a)$, that is,

$(a+b)(b+c)(c+a)\ge 8abc.$

Example 8. a, b, $c>0$. Show that $(\frac{a}{b})^3+(\frac{b}{c})^3+(\frac{c}{a})^3\ge\frac{a^3+b^3+c^3}{abc}$.

Solution:

Method 1:

The original inequality can be written as $(\frac{a}{b})^3+(\frac{b}{c})^3+(\frac{c}{a})^3\ge\frac{a^2}{bc}+\frac{b^2}{ac}+\frac{c^2}{ab}$.

We have the following three similarly ordered sequences:

$\frac{a}{b}, \frac{b}{c}, \frac{c}{a}$

$\frac{a}{b}, \frac{b}{c}, \frac{c}{a}$

$\frac{a}{b}, \frac{b}{c}, \frac{c}{a}$

By the rearrangement inequality, we have

$$\begin{bmatrix} \frac{a}{b} & \frac{b}{c} & \frac{c}{a} \\ \frac{a}{b} & \frac{b}{c} & \frac{c}{a} \\ \frac{a}{b} & \frac{b}{c} & \frac{c}{a} \end{bmatrix} \geq \begin{bmatrix} \frac{a}{b} & \frac{b}{c} & \frac{c}{a} \\ \frac{a}{b} & \frac{b}{c} & \frac{c}{a} \\ \frac{b}{c} & \frac{c}{a} & \frac{a}{b} \end{bmatrix}$$

or

$$(\frac{a}{b})^3 + (\frac{b}{c})^3 + (\frac{c}{a})^3 \geq (\frac{a}{b})(\frac{a}{b})(\frac{b}{c}) + (\frac{b}{c})(\frac{b}{c})(\frac{c}{a}) + (\frac{c}{a})(\frac{c}{a})(\frac{a}{b}) = \frac{a^2}{bc} + \frac{b^2}{ac} + \frac{c^2}{ab}.$$

Method 2:

We have the following three similarly ordered sequences:

$\frac{a}{b}, \frac{b}{c}, \frac{c}{a}$

$(\frac{a}{b})^2, (\frac{b}{c})^2, (\frac{c}{a})^2$

By the rearrangement inequality, we have

$$\begin{bmatrix} \frac{a}{b} & \frac{b}{c} & \frac{c}{a} \\ (\frac{a}{b})^2 & (\frac{b}{c})^2 & (\frac{c}{a})^2 \end{bmatrix} \geq \begin{bmatrix} \frac{a}{b} & \frac{b}{c} & \frac{c}{a} \\ (\frac{c}{a})^2 & (\frac{a}{b})^2 & (\frac{b}{c})^2 \end{bmatrix}$$

$$(\frac{a}{b})^3 + (\frac{b}{c})^3 + (\frac{c}{a})^3 \geq (\frac{a}{b})(\frac{c}{a})^2 + (\frac{b}{c})(\frac{a}{b})^2 + (\frac{c}{a})(\frac{b}{c})^2 = \frac{c^2}{ab} + \frac{a^2}{bc} + \frac{b^2}{ac}.$$

Method 3:

The original inequality can be written as $(\frac{a}{b})^3 + (\frac{b}{c})^3 + (\frac{c}{a})^3 \geq \frac{a^2}{bc} + \frac{b^2}{ac} + \frac{c^2}{ab}$.

Let $x = \frac{a}{b}, y = \frac{b}{c}, z = \frac{c}{a}$.

The inequality becomes $x^3 + y^3 + z^3 \ge \frac{x}{z} + \frac{y}{x} + \frac{z}{y}$, with $xyz = 1$.

or $x^3 + y^3 + z^3 \ge \frac{x(xyz)}{z} + \frac{y(xyz)}{x} + \frac{z(xyz)}{y} = x^2y + y^2z + z^2x$ (1)

For the following similarly ordered sequences,

x, y, z

$x^2, y^2 z^2$

By the rearrangement inequality, we have

$x \quad y \quad z \qquad x \quad y \quad z \quad x$

$x^2 \quad y^2 \quad z^2 \qquad x^2 \quad y^2 \quad z^2 \quad x^2$

$x^3 + y^3 + z^3 \ge x^2y + y^2z + z^2x$. QED.

Method 4:

The original inequality can be written as $(\frac{a}{b})^3 + (\frac{b}{c})^3 + (\frac{c}{a})^3 \ge \frac{a^2}{bc} + \frac{b^2}{ac} + \frac{c^2}{ab}$.

Let $x = \frac{a}{b}, y = \frac{b}{c}, z = \frac{c}{a}$.

The inequality becomes $x^3 + y^3 + z^3 \ge \frac{x}{z} + \frac{y}{x} + \frac{z}{y}$, with $xyz = 1$.

or $x^3 + y^3 + z^3 \ge \frac{x(xyz)}{z} + \frac{y(xyz)}{x} + \frac{z(xyz)}{y} = x^2y + y^2z + z^2x$ (1)

By AM-GM, we have

$x^3 + y^3 + z^3 \ge 3x^2y$ (2)

$x^3 + y^3 + z^3 \ge 3y^2z$ (3)

$x^3 + y^3 + z^3 \ge 3z^2x$ (4)

(1) + (2) + (3): $3(x^3 + y^3 + z^3) \ge 3(x^2y + y^2z + z^2x)$, that is,

$x^3 + y^3 + z^3 \ge x^2y + y^2z + z^2x$. QED.

Example 9. Let a, b be positive numbers with $ab = 1$, prove that

$\frac{a}{b} + \frac{b}{a} \ge a + b$.

Solution:

We have the following two similarly ordered sequences:

$(\sqrt[4]{(\frac{a}{b})^3}, \sqrt[4]{(\frac{b}{a})^3})$

$(\sqrt[4]{\frac{a}{b}}, \sqrt[4]{\frac{b}{a}},),$

By the rearrangement inequality, we have

$$\begin{array}{cccc} \sqrt[4]{(\frac{a}{b})^3} & \sqrt[4]{(\frac{b}{a})^3} & \sqrt[4]{(\frac{a}{b})^3} & \sqrt[4]{(\frac{b}{a})^3} \\ \downarrow & \downarrow & \times & \\ \sqrt[4]{\frac{a}{b}} & \sqrt[4]{\frac{b}{a}} & \sqrt[4]{\frac{a}{b}} & \sqrt[4]{\frac{b}{a}} \end{array}$$

$$\frac{a}{b}+\frac{b}{a} \geq \sqrt[4]{(\frac{a}{b})^3} \cdot \sqrt[4]{\frac{b}{a}} + \sqrt[4]{(\frac{b}{a})^3} \cdot \sqrt[4]{\frac{a}{a}}$$

$$= \sqrt[4]{\frac{a^2}{b^2}} + \sqrt[4]{\frac{b^2}{a^2}} = \sqrt[4]{\frac{a^2(a^2b^2)}{b^2}} + \sqrt[4]{\frac{b^2(a^2b^2)}{a^2}}$$

$$= \sqrt[4]{a^4} + \sqrt[4]{b^4} = a + b.$$

Example 10. Show that for real positive numbers a, b, $\frac{a^n+b^n}{a+b} \geq \frac{1}{2}(a^{n-1} + b^{n-1})$.

Solution:

The given inequality can be written as

$2(a^n + b^n) \geq (a^{n-1} + b^{n-1})(a + b)$

or $2(a^n + b^n) \geq a^n + b^n + ba^{n-1} + ab^{n-1}$

or $a^n + b^n \geq ba^{n-1} + ab^{n-1}$

The following two sequences are similarly ordered:

a, b

a^{n-1}, b^{n-1}.

By the rearrangement inequality, we have

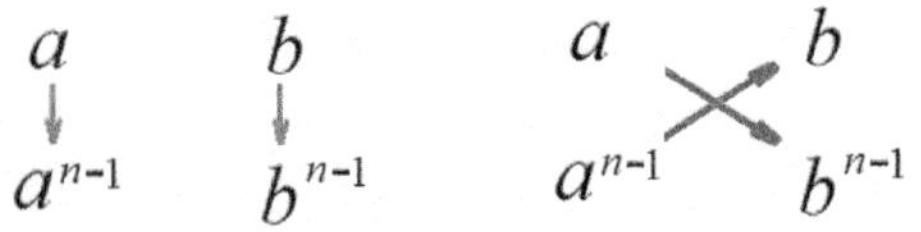

$a \quad b \qquad a \quad b$

$a^{n-1} \quad b^{n-1} \qquad a^{n-1} \quad b^{n-1}$

$a \cdot a^{n-1} + b \cdot b^{n-1} = a^n + b^n \geq a \cdot b^{n-1} + b \cdot a^{n-1} = ba^{n-1} + ab^{n-1}$. QED.

Example 11. Show that for real positive numbers a, b, $2(a^5 + b^5) \geq (a^3 + b^3)(a^2 + b^2)$.

Solution:
The given inequality can be written as $2(a^5 + b^5) \geq a^5 + b^5 + a^2b^3 + b^2a^3$
or $a^5 + b^5 \geq a^2b^3 + b^2a^3$ (1)

We have the following two similarly ordered sequences:
a^2, b^2,
a^3, b^3
By the rearrangement inequality, we have

$a^2 \quad b^2 \qquad a^2 \quad b^2$

$a^3 \quad b^3 \qquad a^3 \quad b^3$

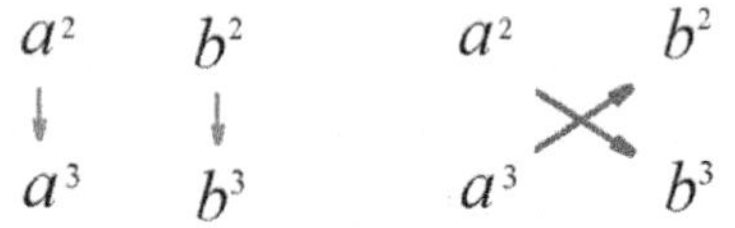

$a^2 \cdot a^3 + b^2 \cdot b^3 = a^5 + b^5 \geq a^2b^3 + a^3b^2$. QED.

Example 12. For nonnegative numbers a, b, c, $3(a^3 + b^3 + c^3) \geq (a + b + c)(a^2 + b^2 + c^2)$

Proof:
We have the following similarly ordered sequences,
$a, \ b, \ c$
$a^2, b^2 \ c^2$

By the rearrangement inequality, we have

$a \quad b \quad c \qquad a \quad b \quad c \quad a$

$a^2 \quad b^2 \quad c^2 \qquad a^2 \quad b^2 \quad c^2 \quad a^2$

$a^3 + b^3 + c^3 \geq a^3 + b^3 + c^3$ (1)

$a^3 + b^3 + c^3 \geq ab^2 + bc^2 + ca^2$ (2)

$$\begin{matrix} a & b & c \\ \downarrow & \downarrow & \downarrow \\ a^2 & b^2 & c^2 \end{matrix} \qquad \begin{matrix} & a & & b & & c & & a \\ a^2 & \nearrow & b^2 & \nearrow & c^2 & \nearrow & a^2 & \end{matrix}$$

$a^3 + b^3 + c^3 \geq a^2b + b^2c + c^2a$ (3)

(1) + (2) + (3):

$3(a^3 + b^3 + c^3) \geq a^3 + b^3 + c^3 + ab^2 + bc^2 + ca^2 + a^2b + b^2c + c^2a$

$= (a^3 + ab^2 + c^2a) + (b^3 + bc^2 + a^2b) + (c^3 + b^2c + ca^2)$

$= a(a^2 + b^2 + c^2) + b(b^2 + c^2 + a^2) + c(c^2 + b^2 + a^2)$

$= (a + b + c)(a^2 + b^2 + c^2)$. QED.

Example 13. Prove that when a, b and c are real numbers,

$$a^4 + b^4 + c^4 \geq a^2b^2 + b^2c^2 + c^2a^2$$

Solution:

For the following similarly ordered sequences,

a^2, b^2, c^2

a^2, b^2, c^2

By the rearrangement inequality, we have

$$\begin{matrix} a^2 & b^2 & c^2 \\ \downarrow & \downarrow & \downarrow \\ a^2 & b^2 & c^2 \end{matrix} \qquad \begin{matrix} a^2 & & b^2 & & c^2 & & a^2 \\ & \searrow & & \searrow & & \searrow & \\ a^2 & & b^2 & & c^2 & & a^2 \end{matrix}$$

$a^2 \cdot a^2 + b^2 \cdot b^2 + c^2 \cdot c^2 \geq a^2 \cdot b^2 + b^2 \cdot c^2 + c^2 \cdot a^2$. QED.

Example 14. Show that when a, b and c are positive real numbers, $\frac{a}{b} + \frac{c}{a} + \frac{b}{c} \geq 3$

Solution:

For the following similarly ordered sequences,

a, b, c

$\frac{1}{c}, \frac{1}{b}, \frac{1}{a}$

by the rearrangement inequality, we have

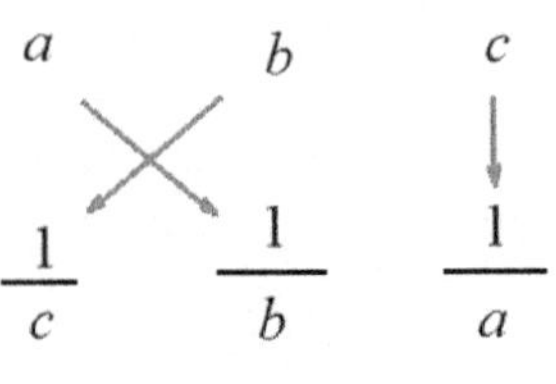

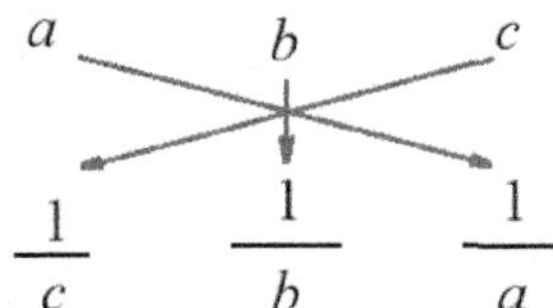

$\frac{a}{b} + \frac{c}{a} + \frac{b}{c} \geq \frac{a}{a} + \frac{b}{b} + \frac{c}{c} = 3$. QED.

Example 15. Let $a, b, c \in R$ such that $a + b + c \geq abc$. Prove the inequality $a^2 + b^2 + c^2 \geq \sqrt{3}abc$.

Proof:

Method 1:

Squaring both sides of the given inequality, we get

$$(a^2 + b^2 + c^2)^2 = a^4 + b^4 + c^4 + 2a^2b^2 + 2b^2c^2 + 2c^2a^2 \geq 3a^2b^2c^2 \quad (1)$$

For the following two sequences,

$a^2, b^2\ c^2$

$a^2, b^2\ c^2$

by the rearrangement inequality, we have

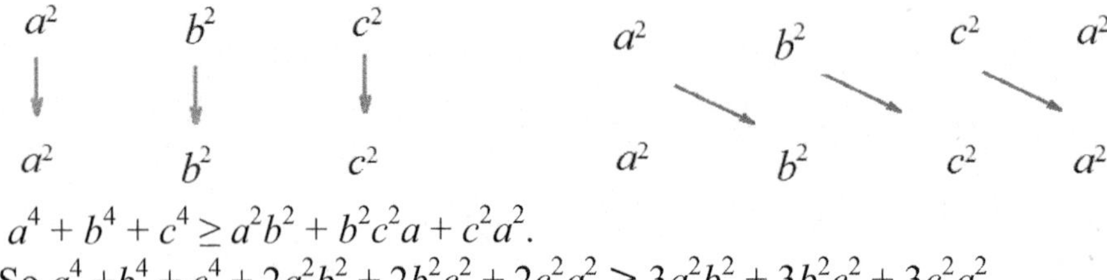

$a^4 + b^4 + c^4 \geq a^2b^2 + b^2c^2a + c^2a^2$.

So $a^4 + b^4 + c^4 + 2a^2b^2 + 2b^2c^2 + 2c^2a^2 \geq 3a^2b^2 + 3b^2c^2 + 3c^2a^2$.

Now we only need to prove

$3a^2b^2 + 3b^2c^2 + 3c^2a^2 \geq 3a^2b^2c^2$

or $a^2b^2 + b^2c^2 + c^2a^2 \geq a^2b^2c^2$.

For the following similarly ordered sequences,
ab, ac, bc
ab, ac, bc
by the rearrangement inequality, we have

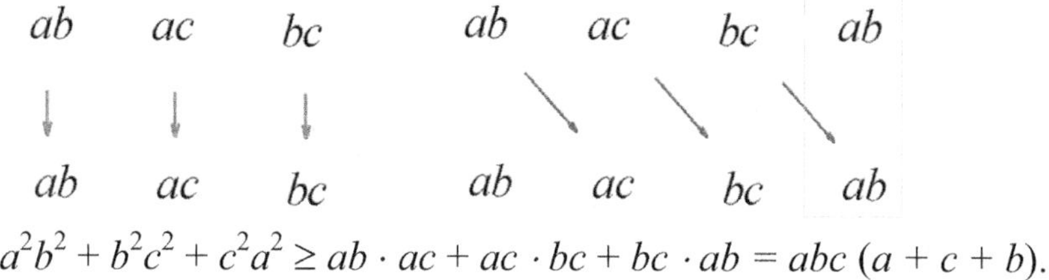

$a^2b^2 + b^2c^2 + c^2a^2 \geq ab \cdot ac + ac \cdot bc + bc \cdot ab = abc\,(a + c + b)$.

Since $a + b + c \geq abc$, $a^2b^2 + b^2c^2 + c^2a^2 \geq a^2b^2c^2$.

Therefore, $(a^2 + b^2 + c^2)^2 \geq 3a^2b^2c^2$
That is, $a^2 + b^2 + c^2 \geq \sqrt{3}abc$.

Method 2:
We have
$(a^2 + b^2 + c^2)^2 = a^4 + b^4 + c^4 + 2a^2b^2 + 2b^2c^2 + 2c^2a^2$
$= a^4 + b^4 + c^4 + a^2(b^2 + c^2) + b^2(c^2 + a^2) + c^2(a^2 + b^2)$ (1)

We know that $a^4 + b^4 + c^4 \geq abc(a + b + c)$ (2)

Also $b^2 + c^2 \geq 2bc$, $c^2 + a^2 \geq 2ca$, $a^2 + b^2 \geq 2ab$ (3)

Now by (1), (2) and (3) we deduce
$(a^2 + b^2 + c^2)^2 \geq abc(a + b + c) + 2a^2bc + 2b^2ac + 2c^2ab$
$= abc(a + b + c) + 2abc(a + b + c) = 3abc(a + b + c)$ (4)

Since $a + b + c \geq abc$ in (4) we have
$(a^2 + b^2 + c^2)^2 \geq 3abc(a + b + c) \geq 3(abc)^2$,
i.e. $a^2 + b^2 + c^2 \geq \sqrt{3}abc$.
Equality occurs if and only if $a = b = c = \sqrt{3}$.

Example 17. Let a, b, c be positive real numbers. Prove that
$\frac{a^3}{c^2} + \frac{b^3}{a^2} + \frac{c^3}{b^2} \geq a + b + c$.

Proof:
The expression is a not symmetric function of a, b, and c. However, we have the following similarly ordered sequences:
a^3, b^3, c^3.
$\frac{1}{c^2}, \frac{1}{b^2}, \frac{1}{a^2}$

By the rearrangement inequality, we have

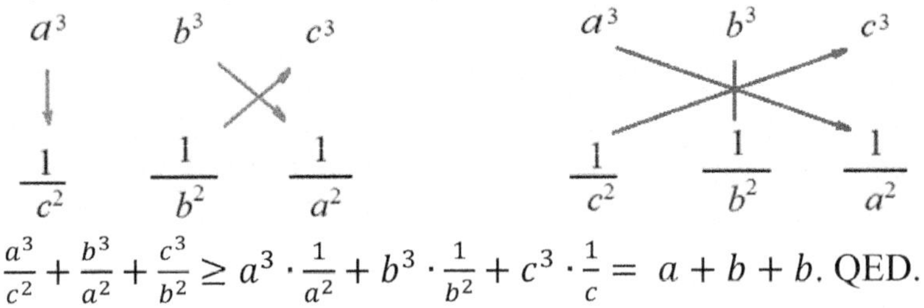

$\frac{a^3}{c^2} + \frac{b^3}{a^2} + \frac{c^3}{b^2} \geq a^3 \cdot \frac{1}{a^2} + b^3 \cdot \frac{1}{b^2} + c^3 \cdot \frac{1}{c} = a + b + b$. QED.

Example 18. Show that for positive real numbers a, b, c, $\frac{a^2+c^2}{b} + \frac{b^2+a^2}{c} + \frac{c^2+a^2}{a} \geq 2(a + b + c)$.

Solution:
The expression $\frac{a^2+c^2}{b} + \frac{b^2+a^2}{c} + \frac{c^2+a^2}{a}$ is neither a symmetric nor cyclic of a, b and c.

However, we are still able to use the rearrangement inequality to solve the problem since we can have the following similarly ordered sequences:
a^2, b^2, c^2
$\frac{1}{c}, \frac{1}{b}, \frac{1}{a}$.

By the rearrangement inequality,

$a^2 \quad b^2 \quad c^2 \qquad\qquad a^2 \quad b^2 \quad c^2$

$\frac{1}{c} \quad \frac{1}{b} \quad \frac{1}{a} \qquad\qquad \frac{1}{c} \quad \frac{1}{b} \quad \frac{1}{a}$

$$\frac{a^2}{b} + \frac{b^2}{c} + \frac{c^2}{a} \geq \frac{a^2}{a} + \frac{b^2}{b} + \frac{c^2}{c} = (a + b + c) \qquad (1)$$

$a^2 \quad b^2 \quad c^2 \qquad\qquad a^2 \quad b^2 \quad c^2$

$\frac{1}{c} \quad \frac{1}{b} \quad \frac{1}{a} \qquad\qquad \frac{1}{c} \quad \frac{1}{b} \quad \frac{1}{a}$

$$\frac{a^2}{c} + \frac{b^2}{a} + \frac{c^2}{b} \geq \frac{a^2}{a} + \frac{b^2}{b} + \frac{c^2}{c} = (a + b + c) \qquad (2)$$

(1) + (2): $\frac{a^2+c^2}{b} + \frac{b^2+a^2}{c} + \frac{c^2+a^2}{a} \geq 2(a + b + c)$.

Example 19. *a*, *b*, *c* $\in R$. Prove that $\frac{a^2b}{c} + \frac{b^2c}{a} + \frac{c^2a}{b} \geq ab + bc + ca$.

Solution:

We can have the following similarly ordered sequences:

a^2b^2, a^2c^2, b^2c^2

$\frac{1}{bc}, \frac{1}{ac}, \frac{1}{ab}$.

By the rearrangement inequality,

$a^2b^2 \quad a^2c^2 \quad b^2c^2 \qquad\qquad a^2b^2 \quad a^2c^2 \quad b^2c^2$

$\frac{1}{bc} \quad \frac{1}{ac} \quad \frac{1}{ab} \qquad\qquad \frac{1}{bc} \quad \frac{1}{ac} \quad \frac{1}{ab}$

$$a^2b^2 \cdot \frac{1}{bc} + a^2c^2 \cdot \frac{1}{ab} + b^2c^2 \cdot \frac{1}{ac} = \frac{a^2b}{c} + \frac{b^2c}{a} + \frac{c^2a}{b}$$

$$\geq a^2b^2 \cdot \frac{1}{ab} + a^2c^2 \cdot \frac{1}{ac} + b^2c^2 \cdot \frac{1}{bc} = ab + ac + bc\,.$$

Example 20. $a, b, c \in R$. Prove that $\frac{a^3b^2}{c}+\frac{b^3c^2}{a}+\frac{c^3a^2}{b} \geq a^2b^2+b^2c^2+c^2a^2$.

Solution:

We can have the following similarly ordered sequences:

a^3b^3, a^3c^3, b^3c^3

$\frac{1}{bc}, \frac{1}{ac}, \frac{1}{ab}$.

By the rearrangement inequality,

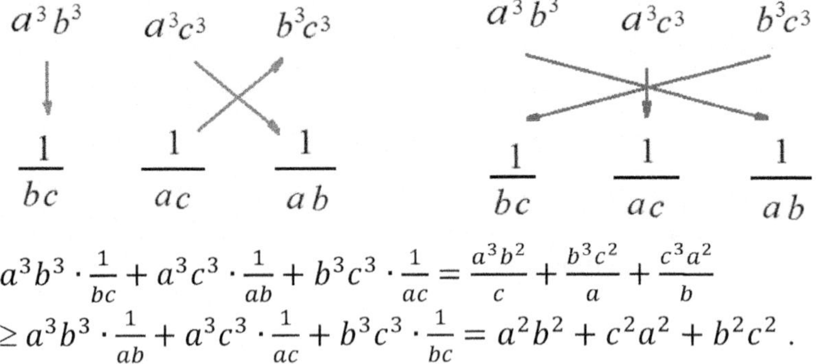

$$a^3b^3\cdot\frac{1}{bc}+a^3c^3\cdot\frac{1}{ab}+b^3c^3\cdot\frac{1}{ac}=\frac{a^3b^2}{c}+\frac{b^3c^2}{a}+\frac{c^3a^2}{b}$$

$$\geq a^3b^3\cdot\frac{1}{ab}+a^3c^3\cdot\frac{1}{ac}+b^3c^3\cdot\frac{1}{bc}=a^2b^2+c^2a^2+b^2c^2.$$

Example 21. Let a, b, c be positive numbers with $abc = 1$, prove that $\frac{a}{b}+\frac{b}{c}+\frac{c}{a} \geq a+b+c$.

Solution:

Method 1:

We have the following two similarly ordered sequences:

$(\sqrt[3]{(\frac{a}{b})^2}, \sqrt[3]{(\frac{b}{c})^2}, \sqrt[3]{(\frac{c}{a})^2})$

$(\sqrt[3]{\frac{a}{b}}, \sqrt[3]{\frac{b}{c}}, \sqrt[3]{\frac{c}{a}})$

By the rearrangement inequality, we have

$$\sqrt[3]{(\frac{a}{b})^2} \quad \sqrt[3]{(\frac{b}{c})^2} \quad \sqrt[3]{(\frac{c}{a})^2} \qquad \sqrt[3]{(\frac{a}{b})^2} \quad \sqrt[3]{(\frac{b}{c})^2} \quad \sqrt[3]{(\frac{c}{a})^2} \quad \sqrt[3]{(\frac{a}{b})^2}$$

$$\sqrt[3]{\frac{a}{b}} \quad \sqrt[3]{\frac{b}{c}} \quad \sqrt[3]{\frac{c}{a}} \qquad \sqrt[3]{\frac{a}{b}} \quad \sqrt[3]{\frac{b}{c}} \quad \sqrt[3]{\frac{c}{a}} \quad \sqrt[3]{\frac{a}{b}}$$

$$\frac{a}{b}+\frac{b}{c}+\frac{c}{a} \ge \sqrt[3]{(\frac{a}{b})^2}\cdot\sqrt[3]{\frac{b}{c}} + \sqrt[3]{(\frac{b}{c})^2}\cdot\sqrt[3]{\frac{c}{a}} + \sqrt[3]{(\frac{c}{a})^2}\cdot\sqrt[3]{\frac{a}{b}}$$

$$= \sqrt[3]{\frac{a^2}{bc}} + \sqrt[3]{\frac{b^2}{ac}} + \sqrt[3]{\frac{c^2}{ab}} = \sqrt[3]{\frac{abc\cdot a^2}{bc}} + \sqrt[3]{\frac{abc\cdot b^2}{ac}} + \sqrt[3]{\frac{abc\cdot c^2}{ab}}$$

$$= \sqrt[3]{a^3} + \sqrt[3]{b^3} + \sqrt[3]{c^3} = a + b + c.$$

Method 2:

By AM-GM, we have

$$\frac{1}{3}\left(\frac{a}{b}+\frac{a}{b}+\frac{b}{c}\right) \ge \sqrt[3]{\frac{a}{b}\cdot\frac{a}{b}\cdot\frac{b}{c}} = \sqrt[3]{\frac{a^2}{bc}} = \sqrt[3]{\frac{abc\cdot a^2}{bc}} = \sqrt[3]{a^3} = a \qquad (1)$$

Similarly,

$$\frac{1}{3}\left(\frac{b}{c}+\frac{b}{c}+\frac{c}{a}\right) \ge b \qquad (2)$$

$$\frac{1}{3}\left(\frac{c}{a}+\frac{c}{a}+\frac{a}{b}\right) \ge c \qquad (3)$$

(1) + (2) + (3):

$$\frac{a}{b}+\frac{b}{c}+\frac{c}{a} \ge a + b + c.$$

CHAPTER 2. PROBLEMS

Problem 1. a, b are positive real numbers. Show that $a + b \geq 2\sqrt{ab}$.

Problem 2. Show that if both a and b are positive, then $\frac{a}{b} + \frac{b}{a} \geq 2$.

Problem 3. Prove that if a, b, c are positive real numbers, then $a^3 + b^3 + c^3 \geq a^2b + b^2c + c^2a$.

Problem 4. Prove that for all positive real numbers a, b, $\frac{a^3}{b} + \frac{b^3}{a} \geq a^2 + b^2$.

Problem 5. If $a, b, c \geq 0$, show that $a^5 + b^5 + c^5 \geq abc(ab + bc + ca)$.

Problem 6. If $a, b, c, d \geq 0$, show that $a^4 + b^4 + c^4 + d^4 \geq 4abcd$.

Problem 7. Given that a, b, c are positive real numbers, prove $2(a^3 + b^3 + c^3) \geq a^2(b + c) + b^2(a + c) + c^2(a + b)$.

Problem 8. Let a, b be positive numbers with $ab = 1$, prove that $a^2 + b^2 \geq a + b$.

Problem 9. Show that for real positive numbers $a, b, n, k, n > k$, $a^n + b^n \geq a^{n-k}b^k + a^k b^{n-k}$.

Problem 10. Show that for real positive numbers a, b, $a^9 + b^9 \geq a^2b^2(a^5 + b^5)$.

Problem 11. For nonnegative numbers a, b, c, show that $2(a^3 + b^3 + c^3) \geq ab\,(a + b) + bc\,(b + c) + ca(c + a)$.

Problem 12. Show that for real numbersa, b, c, we have $a^4 + b^4 + c^4 \geq a^2bc + b^2ac + c^2ab$.

Problem 13. Show that when a, b and c are real numbers, $a^2b^2 + b^2c^2 + c^2a^2 \geq abc$ $(a + c + b)$.

Problem 14. (Titu Andreescu) Show that for real positive numbers a, b, c ,
$\frac{a^2}{b^2} + \frac{b^2}{c^2} + \frac{c^2}{a^2} \geq \frac{a}{c} + \frac{c}{b} + \frac{b}{a}$.

Problem 15. Let a, b, c be positive real numbers. Prove that $\frac{a^2}{b} + \frac{b^2}{c} + \frac{c^2}{a}$ $\geq a + b + c$.

Problem 16. Let a, b, c be positive real numbers. Prove that
$\frac{a^4}{b^2} + \frac{b^4}{c^2} + \frac{c^4}{a^2} \geq a^2 + b^2 + c^2$.

Problem 17. Show that $ab + bc + ca \leq \frac{1}{3}$. a, b, c are positive with $a + b + c =$ 1.

Problem 18. a, b, c $\in R$. Prove that $\frac{a^2c}{b} + \frac{b^2a}{c} + \frac{c^2b}{a} \geq ab + bc + ca$.

Problem 19. a, b, c $\in R$. Prove that $\frac{a^3c^2}{b} + \frac{b^3a^2}{c} + \frac{c^3b^2}{a} \geq a^2b^2 + b^2c^2 + c^2a^2$.

Problem 20. Let a, b, c be positive real numbers with $abc = 1$. Prove that
$\frac{a^2}{b^2} + \frac{b^2}{c^2} + \frac{c^2}{a^2} \geq a^2 + b^2 + c^2$.

CHAPTER 2. SOLUTIONS

Problem 1. Solution:

We have the following two similarly ordered sequences:

$\sqrt{a}, \sqrt{b}$

$\sqrt{a}, \sqrt{b}$

By the rearrangement inequality, we have

$$\begin{matrix} \sqrt{a} & \sqrt{b} \\ \downarrow & \downarrow \\ \sqrt{a} & \sqrt{b} \end{matrix} \qquad \begin{matrix} \sqrt{a} & & \sqrt{b} \\ & \times & \\ \sqrt{a} & & \sqrt{b} \end{matrix}$$

or $\begin{bmatrix} \sqrt{a} & \sqrt{b} \\ \sqrt{a} & \sqrt{b} \end{bmatrix} \geq \begin{bmatrix} \sqrt{a} & \sqrt{b} \\ \sqrt{b} & \sqrt{a} \end{bmatrix}$.

$\sqrt{a} \cdot \sqrt{a} + \sqrt{b} \cdot \sqrt{b} = a + b \geq \sqrt{a} \cdot \sqrt{b} + \sqrt{a} \cdot \sqrt{b} = 2\sqrt{ab}$,

where both a and b are nonnegative real numbers and equality occurs if and only if $a = b$.

Problem 2. Solution:

If $a \leq b$, then $\frac{1}{b} \leq \frac{1}{a}$; If $a \geq b$, then $\frac{1}{b} \geq \frac{1}{a}$. Thus the following two sequences are similarly ordered:

a, b

$\frac{1}{b}, \frac{1}{a}$

By the rearrangement inequality, we have

$$\begin{matrix} a & b \\ \downarrow & \downarrow \\ \frac{1}{b} & \frac{1}{a} \end{matrix} \qquad \begin{matrix} a & & b \\ & \times & \\ \frac{1}{b} & & \frac{1}{a} \end{matrix}$$

or $\begin{bmatrix} a & b \\ \frac{1}{b} & \frac{1}{a} \end{bmatrix} \geq \begin{bmatrix} a & b \\ \frac{1}{a} & \frac{1}{b} \end{bmatrix}$.

$a \cdot \frac{1}{b} + b \cdot \frac{1}{a} = \frac{a}{b} + \frac{b}{a} \geq a \cdot \frac{1}{a} + b \cdot \frac{1}{b} = 1 + 1 = 2.$

Problem 3. Solution:

For the following two similarly ordered sequences,

a, b, c

$a^2, b^2\ c^2$

By the rearrangement inequality, we have

$$\begin{matrix} a & b & c \\ \downarrow & \downarrow & \downarrow \\ a^2 & b^2 & c^2 \end{matrix} \qquad \begin{matrix} a & b & c & a \\ \nearrow & \nearrow & \nearrow & \\ a^2 & b^2 & c^2 & a^2 \end{matrix}$$

$a^3 + b^3 + c^3 \geq a^2b + b^2c + c^2a.$

Problem 4. Solution:

Method 1:

Since the expression is a symmetric function of a, b, and c, we can assume, without loss of generality, that $a \leq b$, $a^3 \leq b^3$, and $\frac{1}{b} \leq \frac{1}{a}$.

Then we have the following two similarly ordered sequences:

$a^3, b^3,$

$\frac{1}{b}, \frac{1}{a}$

By the rearrangement inequality, we have

$$\begin{matrix} a^3 & b^3 \\ \downarrow & \downarrow \\ \frac{1}{b} & \frac{1}{a} \end{matrix} \qquad \begin{matrix} a^3 & & b^3 \\ & \times & \\ \frac{1}{b} & & \frac{1}{a} \end{matrix}$$

$\frac{a^3}{b} + \frac{b^3}{a} \geq a^3 \cdot \frac{1}{a} + b^3 \cdot \frac{1}{b} = a^2 + b^2.$

Problem 5. Proof:

For the following similarly ordered sequences,

$a, \ b, \ c$

$a^2, b^2\ c^2$

$a^2, b^2\ c^2$

By the rearrangement inequality, we have

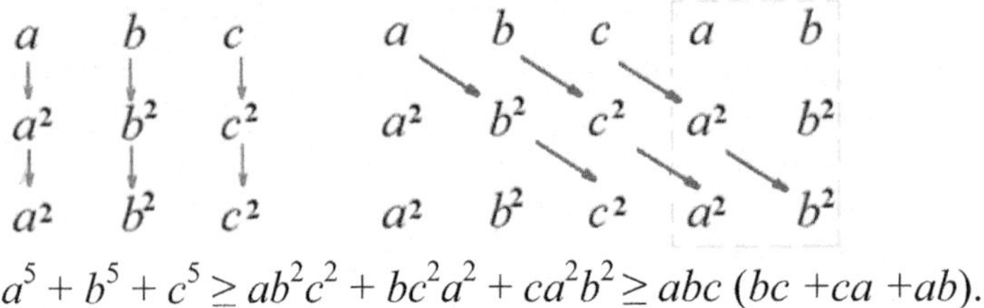

$a^5 + b^5 + c^5 \ge ab^2c^2 + bc^2a^2 + ca^2b^2 \ge abc\ (bc + ca + ab)$.

Problem 6. Solution:

For the following similarly ordered sequences,

a, b, c

a, b, c

a, b, c

by the shoelace inequality, we have

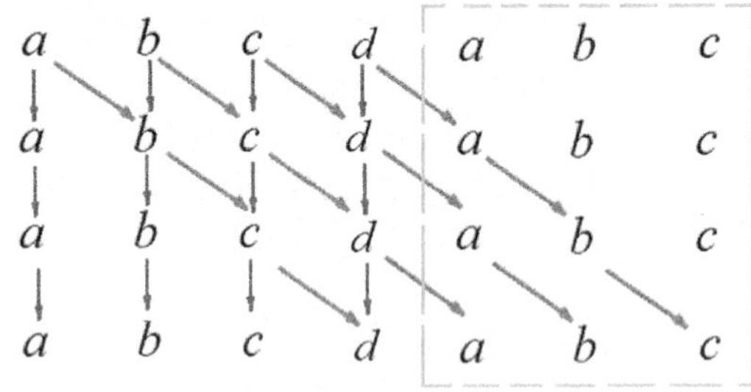

$a^4 + b^4 + c^4 + d^4 \ge 4abcd$.

Problem 7. Solution:

We have the following two similarly ordered sequences:

a, b, c.

a^2, b^2, c^2.

By the rearrangement inequality, we have

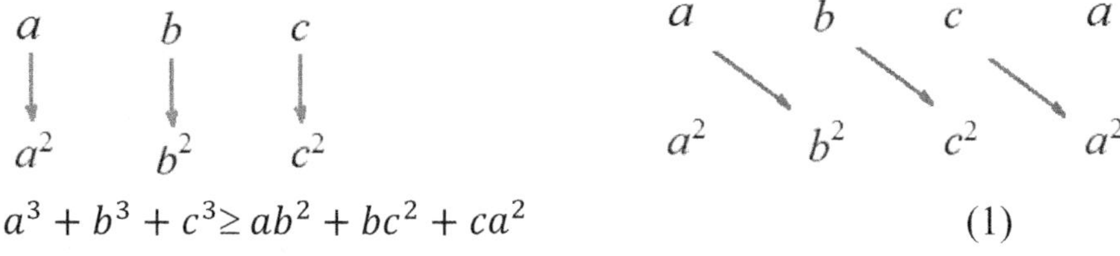

$a^3 + b^3 + c^3 \geq ab^2 + bc^2 + ca^2$ (1)

a b c a b c a

a^2 b^2 c^2 a^2 b^2 c^2 a^2

$a^3 + b^3 + c^3 \geq a^2b + b^2c + c^2a$ (2)

(1) + (2): $2(a^3 + b^3 + c^3) \geq a^2(b + c) + b^2(a + c) + c^2(a + b)$.

Problem 8. Solution:

Since $ab = 1$, we have $a = \frac{1}{b}$ and $b = \frac{1}{a}$.

The given inequality can then be written as

$a(\frac{1}{b}) + b(\frac{1}{a}) \geq a + b$ or $\frac{a}{b} + \frac{b}{a} \geq a + b$.

We have the following two similarly ordered sequences:

$(\sqrt[4]{(\frac{a}{b})^3}, \sqrt[4]{(\frac{b}{a})^3})$

$(\sqrt[4]{\frac{a}{b}}, \sqrt[4]{\frac{b}{a}})$

By the rearrangement inequality, we have

$$\sqrt[4]{\left(\frac{a}{b}\right)^3} \quad \sqrt[4]{\left(\frac{b}{a}\right)^3} \qquad\qquad \sqrt[4]{\left(\frac{a}{b}\right)^3} \quad \sqrt[4]{\left(\frac{b}{a}\right)^3}$$

$$\downarrow \qquad \downarrow \qquad\qquad \times$$

$$\sqrt[4]{\frac{a}{b}} \quad \sqrt[4]{\frac{b}{a}} \qquad\qquad \sqrt[4]{\frac{a}{b}} \quad \sqrt[4]{\frac{b}{a}}$$

$\frac{a}{b}+\frac{b}{a} \geq \sqrt[4]{\left(\frac{a}{b}\right)^3} \cdot \sqrt[4]{\frac{b}{a}}+\sqrt[4]{\left(\frac{b}{a}\right)^3} \cdot \sqrt[4]{\frac{a}{a}}$

$=\sqrt[4]{\frac{a^2}{b^2}}+\sqrt[4]{\frac{b^2}{a^2}}=\sqrt[4]{\frac{a^2(a^2b^2)}{b^2}}+\sqrt[4]{\frac{b^2(a^2b^2)}{a^2}}$

$=\sqrt[4]{a^4}+\sqrt[4]{b^4}=a+b$. QED.

Problem 9. Solution:

The following two sequences are similarly ordered:

a, b

a^{n-1}, b^{n-1}.

By the rearrangement inequality, we have

$$a^k \quad b^k \qquad\qquad a^k \quad b^k$$

$$\downarrow \qquad \downarrow \qquad\qquad \times$$

$$a^{n-k} \quad b^{n-k} \qquad\qquad a^{n-k} \quad b^{n-k}$$

$a^n \cdot a^{n-k}+b^n \cdot b^{n-k} \geq a^k \cdot b^{n-k}+b^k \cdot a^{n-k}$, that is

$a^n+b^n \geq a^{n-k}b^k+a^kb^{n-k}$.

Problem 10. Solution:

The given inequality can be written as

$a^9+b^9 \geq a^7b^2+a^2b^7$ (1)

The following two sequences are similarly ordered:

$a^2, b^2,$
a^7, b^7
By the rearrangement inequality, we have

$$\begin{array}{cc} a^2 & b^2 \\ \downarrow & \downarrow \\ a^7 & b^7 \end{array} \qquad \begin{array}{ccc} a^2 & & b^2 \\ & \times & \\ a^7 & & b^7 \end{array}$$

$a^9 + b^9 \ge a^7b^2 + a^2b^7.$

Problem 11. Proof:
For the following similarly ordered sequences,
$a, \ b, \ c$
$a^2, b^2 \ c^2$

By the rearrangement inequality, we have

$$\begin{array}{ccc} a & b & c \\ \downarrow & \downarrow & \downarrow \\ a^2 & b^2 & c^2 \end{array} \qquad \begin{array}{cccc} a & b & c & a \\ \searrow & \searrow & \searrow & \\ a^2 & b^2 & c^2 & a^2 \end{array}$$

$a^3 + b^3 + c^3 \ge ab^2 + bc^2 + ca^2$ (1)

$$\begin{array}{ccc} a & b & c \\ \downarrow & \downarrow & \downarrow \\ a^2 & b^2 & c^2 \end{array} \qquad \begin{array}{cccc} a & b & c & a \\ \nearrow & \nearrow & \nearrow & \\ a^2 & b^2 & c^2 & a^2 \end{array}$$

$a^3 + b^3 + c^3 \ge a^2b + b^2c + c^2a$ (2)

(1) + (2):
$2(a^3 + b^3 + c^3) \ge ab^2 + a^2b + bc^2 + b^2c + c^2a + ca^2$
$= ab\ (a + b) + bc\ (b + c) + ca(c + a).$ QED.

Problem 12.Proof:
For the following similarly ordered sequences,
$a^2, b^2 \ c^2$
$a^2, b^2 \ c^2$

by the rearrangement inequality, we have

$$\begin{array}{ccc} a^2 & b^2 & c^2 \\ \downarrow & \downarrow & \downarrow \\ a^2 & b^2 & c^2 \end{array} \qquad \begin{array}{cccc} a^2 & b^2 & c^2 & a^2 \\ & \searrow \quad \searrow & \searrow & \\ a^2 & b^2 & c^2 & a^2 \end{array}$$

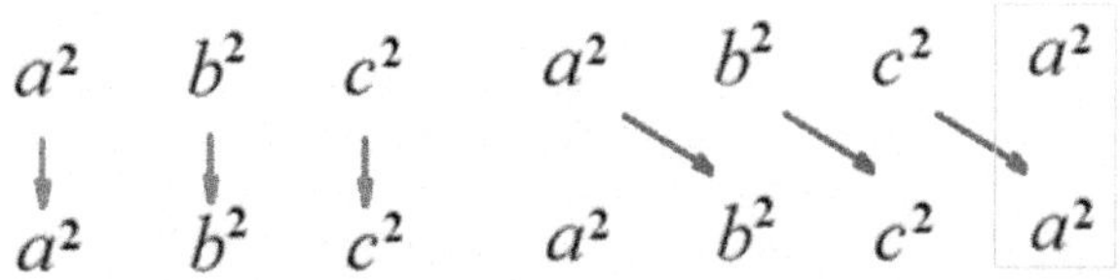

$a^4 + b^4 + c^4 \geq a^2b^2 + b^2c^2a + c^2a^2$

We know that for positive x, y, and z, $x^2 + y^2 + z^2 \geq xy + yz + zx$,

So $a^2b^2 + b^2c^2a + c^2a^2 \geq abbc + bcca + caab = a^2bc + b^2ac + c^2ab$.

Then $a^4 + b^4 + c^4 \geq a^2bc + b^2ac + c^2ab$.

Problem 13. Proof:

For the following similarly ordered sequences,

ab, ac, bc

ab, ac, bc

By the rearrangement inequality, we have

$$\begin{array}{ccc} ab & ac & bc \\ \downarrow & \downarrow & \downarrow \\ ab & ac & bc \end{array} \qquad \begin{array}{cccc} ab & ac & bc & ab \\ & \searrow \quad \searrow & \searrow & \\ ab & ac & bc & ab \end{array}$$

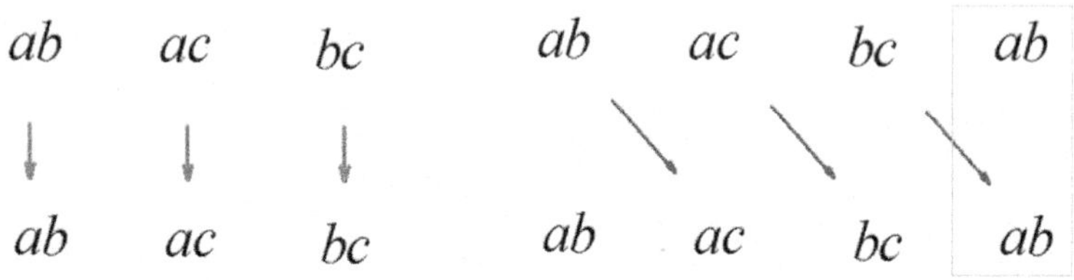

$a^2b^2 + b^2c^2 + c^2a^2 \geq ab \cdot ac + ac \cdot bc + bc \cdot ab = abc\ (a + c + b)$.

Problem 14. Proof:

The following triplets are similarly arranged.

$\frac{a}{b}, \frac{b}{c}, \frac{c}{a}$

$\frac{a}{b}, \frac{b}{c}, \frac{c}{a}$

Hence

$\frac{a}{b}$ $\frac{b}{c}$ $\frac{c}{a}$ $\qquad$ $\frac{a}{b}$ $\frac{b}{c}$ $\frac{c}{a}$ $\frac{a}{b}$

$\frac{a}{b}$ $\frac{b}{c}$ $\frac{c}{a}$ $\qquad$ $\frac{a}{b}$ $\frac{b}{c}$ $\frac{c}{a}$ $\frac{a}{b}$

Then we have

$$\frac{a}{b}\cdot\frac{a}{b}+\frac{b}{c}\cdot\frac{b}{c}+\frac{c}{a}\cdot\frac{c}{a}\ge\frac{a}{b}\cdot\frac{b}{c}+\frac{b}{c}\cdot\frac{c}{a}+\frac{c}{a}\cdot\frac{a}{b}\Rightarrow\frac{a^2}{b^2}+\frac{b^2}{c^2}+\frac{c^2}{a^2}\ge\frac{a}{c}+\frac{c}{b}+\frac{b}{a}.$$

Problem 15. Proof:

Method 1:

For the following similarly sorted sequences,

a^2, b^2, c^2.

$\frac{1}{c}, \frac{1}{b}, \frac{1}{a}$

by the rearrangement inequality, we have

$$\frac{a^2}{b}+\frac{b^2}{c}+\frac{c^2}{a}\ge a^2\cdot\frac{1}{a}+b^2\cdot\frac{1}{b}+c^2\cdot\frac{1}{c}=a+b+c.$$

Equality occurs if and only if $a = b = c$.

Method 2:

From AM-GM, we have

$$\frac{a^2}{b}+b\ge 2\sqrt{\frac{a^2}{b}\cdot b}=2a \qquad (1)$$

Similarly,

$$\frac{b^2}{c}+c\ge 2b \qquad (2)$$

$$\frac{c^2}{a}+a\ge 2c \qquad (3)$$

(1) + (2) + (3):

$$\frac{a^2}{b}+\frac{b^2}{c}+\frac{c^2}{a}+a+b+c \geq 2(a+b+c).$$

i.e.

$$\frac{a^2}{b}+\frac{b^2}{c}+\frac{c^2}{a} \geq a+b+c.$$

Equality occurs if and only if $a = b = c$.

Problem 16. Proof:

The expression is a not symmetric function of a, b, and c. However, we have the following similarly ordered sequences:

a^4, b^4, c^4.

$\frac{1}{c^2}, \frac{1}{b^2}, \frac{1}{a^2}$

By the rearrangement inequality, we have

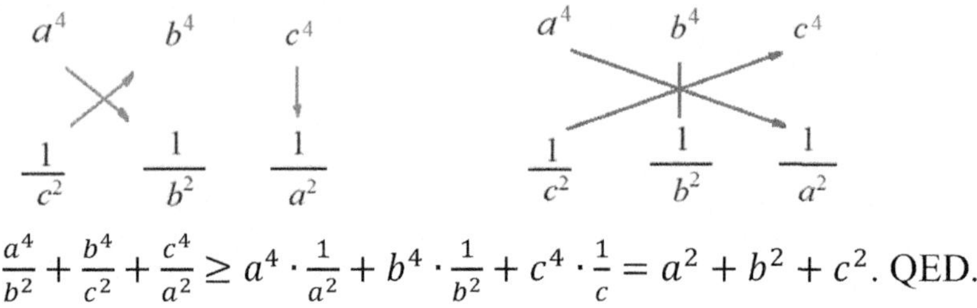

$$\frac{a^4}{b^2}+\frac{b^4}{c^2}+\frac{c^4}{a^2} \geq a^4 \cdot \frac{1}{a^2}+b^4 \cdot \frac{1}{b^2}+c^4 \cdot \frac{1}{c}=a^2+b^2+c^2. \text{ QED.}$$

Problem 17. Proof:

The given inequality can be written as $3(ab+bc+ca) \leq 1$ or

$3(ab+bc+ca) \leq (a+b+c)^2$

or $3(ab+bc+ca) \leq a^2+b^2+c^2+2(ab+bc+ca)$

or $(ab+bc+ca) \leq a^2+b^2+c^2$

For the two similarly sorted sequences

a, b, c

a, b, c

by the rearrangement inequality, we have

$a^2 + b^2 + c^2 \geq ab + bc + ca.$

Problem 18. Solution:

We can have the following similarly ordered sequences:

a^2b^2, a^2c^2, b^2c^2

$\frac{1}{bc}, \frac{1}{ac}, \frac{1}{ab}.$

By the rearrangement inequality,

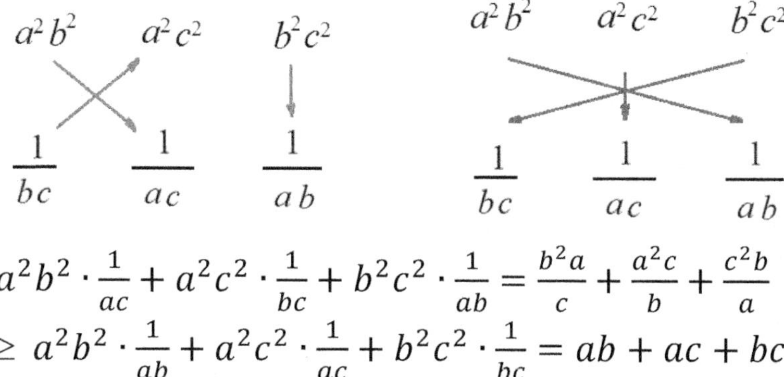

$$a^2b^2 \cdot \frac{1}{ac} + a^2c^2 \cdot \frac{1}{bc} + b^2c^2 \cdot \frac{1}{ab} = \frac{b^2a}{c} + \frac{a^2c}{b} + \frac{c^2b}{a}$$

$$\geq a^2b^2 \cdot \frac{1}{ab} + a^2c^2 \cdot \frac{1}{ac} + b^2c^2 \cdot \frac{1}{bc} = ab + ac + bc$$

Problem 19. Solution:

We can have the following similarly ordered sequences:

a^3b^3, a^3c^3, b^3c^3

$\frac{1}{bc}, \frac{1}{ac}, \frac{1}{ab}.$

By the rearrangement inequality,

$$a^3b^3 \cdot \frac{1}{ac} + a^3c^3 \cdot \frac{1}{bc} + b^3c^3 \cdot \frac{1}{ab} = \frac{a^3c^2}{b} + \frac{b^3a^2}{c} + \frac{c^3b^2}{a}$$

$$\geq a^3b^3 \cdot \frac{1}{ab} + a^3c^3 \cdot \frac{1}{ac} + b^3c^3 \cdot \frac{1}{bc} = a^2b^2 + c^2a^2 + b^2c^2 \quad .$$

Problem 20. Solution:

We have the following two similarly ordered sequences:

$$\left(\sqrt[3]{(\frac{a}{b})^4}, \sqrt[3]{(\frac{b}{c})^4}, \sqrt[3]{(\frac{c}{a})^4}\right)$$

$$\left(\sqrt[3]{(\frac{a}{b})^2}, \sqrt[3]{(\frac{b}{c})^2}, \sqrt[3]{(\frac{c}{a})^2}\right)$$

By the rearrangement inequality, we have

$$\begin{array}{ccc} \sqrt[3]{(\frac{a}{b})^4} & \sqrt[3]{(\frac{b}{c})^4} & \sqrt[3]{(\frac{c}{a})^4} \\ \downarrow & \downarrow & \downarrow \\ \sqrt[3]{(\frac{a}{b})^2} & \sqrt[3]{(\frac{b}{c})^2} & \sqrt[3]{(\frac{c}{a})^2} \end{array} \qquad \begin{array}{cccc} \sqrt[3]{(\frac{a}{b})^4} & \sqrt[3]{(\frac{b}{c})^4} & \sqrt[3]{(\frac{c}{a})^4} & \sqrt[3]{(\frac{a}{b})^4} \\ \searrow & \searrow & \searrow & \\ \sqrt[3]{(\frac{a}{b})^2} & \sqrt[3]{(\frac{b}{c})^2} & \sqrt[3]{(\frac{c}{a})^2} & \sqrt[3]{(\frac{a}{b})^2} \end{array}$$

$$\frac{a^2}{b^2} + \frac{b^2}{c^2} + \frac{c^2}{a^2} \geq \sqrt[3]{(\frac{a}{b})^4} \cdot \sqrt[3]{(\frac{b}{c})^2} + \sqrt[3]{(\frac{b}{c})^4} \cdot \sqrt[3]{(\frac{c}{a})^2}) + \sqrt[3]{(\frac{c}{a})^4} \cdot \sqrt[3]{(\frac{a}{b})^2}$$

$$= \sqrt[3]{\frac{a^4}{b^2c^2}} + \sqrt[3]{\frac{b^4}{a^2c^2}} + \sqrt[3]{\frac{c^4}{b^2a^2}} = = \sqrt[3]{\frac{a^4a^2b^2c^2}{b^2c^2}} + \sqrt[3]{\frac{b^4a^2b^2c^2}{a^2c^2}} + \sqrt[3]{\frac{c^4a^2b^2c^2}{b^2a^2}}$$

$$= \sqrt[3]{a^6} + \sqrt[3]{b^6} + \sqrt[3]{c^6} = a^2 + b^2 + c^2.$$

Chapter 3. Solving Problems with Ordered Variables

In this section, we will solve the inequality problems in which the order of the variables is given. For example, $a \le b \le c$.

Theorem 3.1: If n is a positive integer and $0 \le a \le b \le c \le d$, for the following similarly ordered sequences,

$a,\ b,\ c,\ d$

a^n, b^n, c^n, d^n

we have

$ab^n + bc^n + cd^n + da^n \ge a^n b + b^n c + c^n d + d^n a$.

or

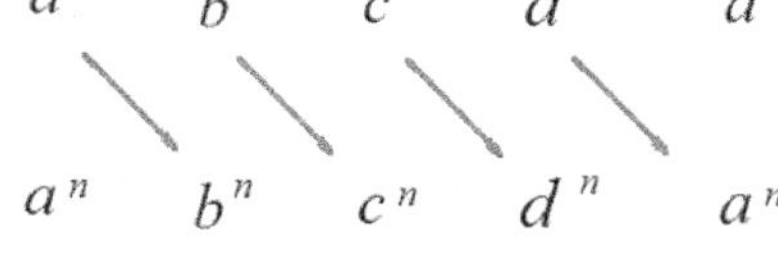
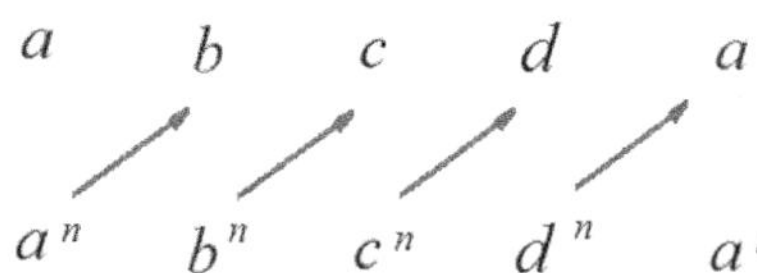

Proof:

The inequality is equivalent to

$$ab^n + bc^n + cd^n + da^n - a^n b - b^n c - c^n d - d^n a \ge 0 \ \Rightarrow$$

$$(ab^n - d^n a) + (bc^n - a^n b) + (cd^n - b^n c) + (da^n - c^n d) \ge 0 \ \Rightarrow$$

$$(d^n - b^n)(c-a) - (c^n - a^n)(d-b) \ge 0 \ \Rightarrow$$

$$(d-b)(c-a)[(d^{n-1} + d^{n-2}b + d^{n-3}b^2 + \ldots + b^{n-1})$$

$$-(c^{n-1} + c^{n-2}a + c^{n-3}a^2 + \ldots + a^{n-1})] \ge 0.$$

The last inequality is certainly true.

For three variable a, b, and c, we have:

Theorem 3.2: If n is a positive integer and $0 \le a \le b \le c$, then

$ab^n + bc^n + ca^n \ge a^n b + b^n c + c^n a$.

Theorem 3.3: If $a \le b \le c, \frac{1}{c} \le \frac{1}{b} \le \frac{1}{a}$, where a, b, c, are real positive numbers, we have $\frac{a}{b}+\frac{b}{c}+\frac{c}{a} \ge \frac{a}{c}+\frac{c}{b}+\frac{b}{a}$,

or

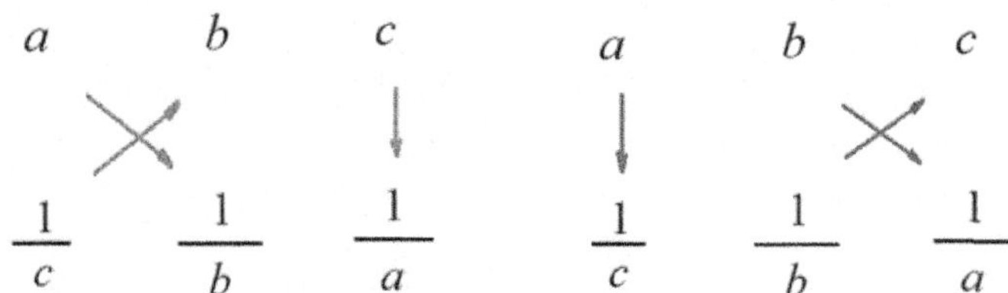

Proof:

$\frac{a}{b}+\frac{b}{c}+\frac{c}{a} \ge \frac{a}{c}+\frac{c}{b}+\frac{b}{a} \quad \Leftrightarrow \quad \frac{a^2c+b^2a+c^2b}{abc} \ge \frac{a^2b+b^2c+c^2a}{abc}$

$\Leftrightarrow \quad a^2c+b^2a+c^2b \ge a^2b+b^2c+c^2a \quad \Leftrightarrow$

$\Leftrightarrow \quad a^2c+b^2a+c^2b - a^2b - b^2c - c^2a \ge 0 \quad \Leftrightarrow$

$(c-a)(b-a)(c-b) \ge 0$

The last inequality is certainly true.

Replace a with a^2, b with b^2, and c with c^2, we have

Theorem 3.4: If $a \le b \le c$, where a, b, c, are real positive numbers, we have

$\frac{a^2}{b^2}+\frac{b^2}{c^2}+\frac{c^2}{a^2} \ge \frac{a^2}{c^2}+\frac{b^2}{a^2}+\frac{c^2}{b^2}$

or

$a^2 \quad b^2 \quad c^2 \qquad a^2 \quad b^2 \quad c^2$

$\frac{1}{c^2} \quad \frac{1}{b^2} \quad \frac{1}{a^2} \qquad \frac{1}{c^2} \quad \frac{1}{b^2} \quad \frac{1}{a^2}$

Theorem 3.5: If $a \le b \le c$, where a, b, c, are real positive numbers, for two ordered sequences, a^2, b^2, c^2 and $\frac{1}{c}, \frac{1}{b}, \frac{1}{a}$, we have $\frac{a^2}{b}+\frac{b^2}{c}+\frac{c^2}{a} \ge \frac{a^2}{c}+\frac{b^2}{a}+\frac{c^2}{b}$

or

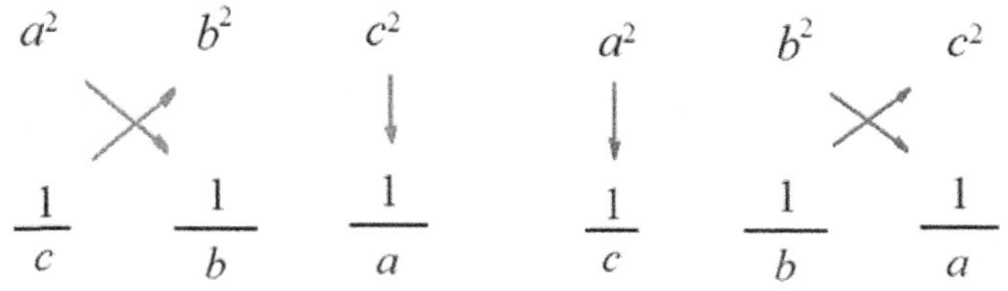

$a^2 \quad b^2 \quad c^2 \qquad a^2 \quad b^2 \quad c^2$

$\frac{1}{c} \quad \frac{1}{b} \quad \frac{1}{a} \qquad \frac{1}{c} \quad \frac{1}{b} \quad \frac{1}{a}$

Proof:

$\frac{a^2}{b}+\frac{b^2}{c}+\frac{c^2}{a}\geq \frac{a^2}{c}+\frac{b^2}{a}+\frac{c^2}{b} \qquad \Leftrightarrow \frac{a^3c+b^3a+c^3b}{abc}\geq \frac{a^3b+b^3c+c^3a}{abc} \qquad \Leftrightarrow$

$a^3c+b^3a+c^3b\geq a^3b+b^3c+c^3a$

$\Leftrightarrow \qquad a^3c+b^3a+c^3b-a^3b-b^3c-c^3a\geq 0$

$\Leftrightarrow \qquad (c-a)(b-a)[(c^2-b^2)+a(c-b)]\geq 0$

The last inequality is certainly true.

Theorem 3.6: If $a \leq b \leq c$, where a, b, c, are real positive numbers, for two similarly sorted sequences, a^3, b^3, c^3 and $\frac{1}{c^2}, \frac{1}{b^2}, \frac{1}{a^2}$, we have $\frac{a^3}{b^2}+\frac{b^3}{c^2}+\frac{c^3}{a^2}\geq \frac{a^3}{c^2}+\frac{b^3}{a^2}+\frac{c^3}{b^2}$

or

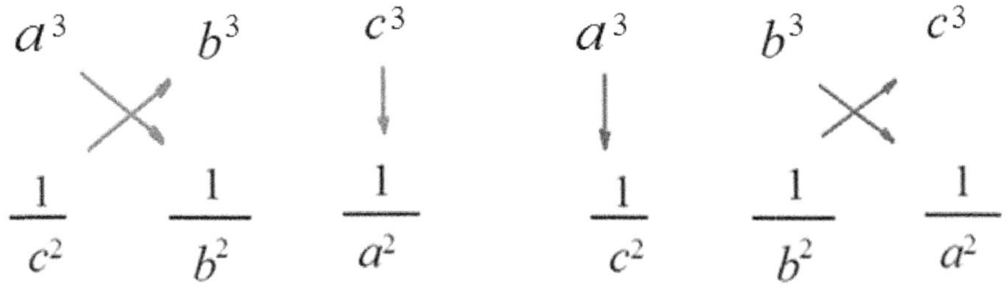

$a^3 \quad b^3 \quad c^3 \qquad a^3 \quad b^3 \quad c^3$

$\frac{1}{c^2} \quad \frac{1}{b^2} \quad \frac{1}{a^2} \qquad \frac{1}{c^2} \quad \frac{1}{b^2} \quad \frac{1}{a^2}$

Proof:

$\frac{a^3}{b^2}+\frac{b^3}{c^2}+\frac{c^3}{a^2}\geq \frac{a^3}{c^2}+\frac{b^3}{a^2}+\frac{c^3}{b^2} \qquad \Leftrightarrow \qquad \frac{a^5c^2+b^5a^2+c^5b^2}{a^2b^2c^2}\geq \frac{a^5b^2+b^5c^2+c^5a^2}{a^2b^2c^2}$

$\Leftrightarrow \qquad a^5c^2+b^5a^2+c^5b^2\geq a^5b^2+b^5c^2+c^5a^2$

$$\Leftrightarrow \quad a^5c^2 + b^5a^2 + c^5b^2 - (a^5b^2 + b^5c^2 + c^5a^2) \ge 0 \Leftrightarrow$$

$(c-a)(b-a)(c-b)(a^3b + ab^3 + a^3c + ac^3 + b^3c + bc^3 + a^2b^2 + b^2c^2 + c^2a^2 + 2a^2bc + 2ab^2c + 2abc^2) \ge 0$

The last inequality is certainly true.

Example 1. If $0 \le a \le b \le c$, show that $ab^2 + bc^2 + ca^2 \ge a^2b + b^2c + c^2a$.

Solution:

We have the following two similarly ordered sequences.

$a,\ b,\ c$

$a^2, b^2\ c^2$

By the rearrangement inequality, we have

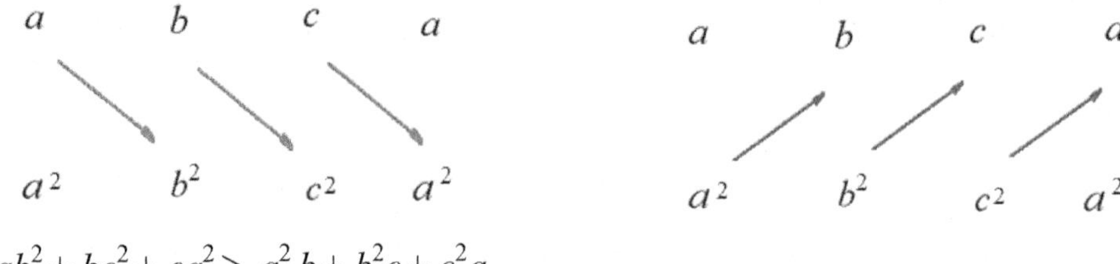

$ab^2 + bc^2 + ca^2 \ge a^2b + b^2c + c^2a$.

Method 2:

$ab^2 + bc^2 + ca^2 \ge a^2b + b^2c + c^2a \quad \Leftrightarrow ab^2 + bc^2 + ca^2 - (a^2b + b^2c + c^2a) \ge 0$

$ab^2 + bc^2 + ca^2 - (a^2b + b^2c + c^2a)$

$= (ab^2 - a^2b) + (bc^2 - c^2a) + (ca^2 - b^2c)$

$= ab(b-a) + c^2(b-a) + c(a^2 - b^2)$

$= (b-a)[ab + c^2 - c(a+b)]$

$= (b-a)[ab - ca + c^2 - cb]$

$= (b-a)[a(b-c) + c(c-b)]$

$= (b-a)(c-b)(c-a) \ge 0$. QED.

Example 2. If $0 \le a \le b \le c \le d$, show that $ab^2 + bc^2 + cd^2 + da^2 \ge a^2 b + b^2c + c^2d + d^2a$.

Solution:

Method 1:

We have the following two similarly ordered sequences.

$a, \ b, c, \ d$

$a^2, b^2 \ c^2, d^2$

By the rearrangement inequality, we have

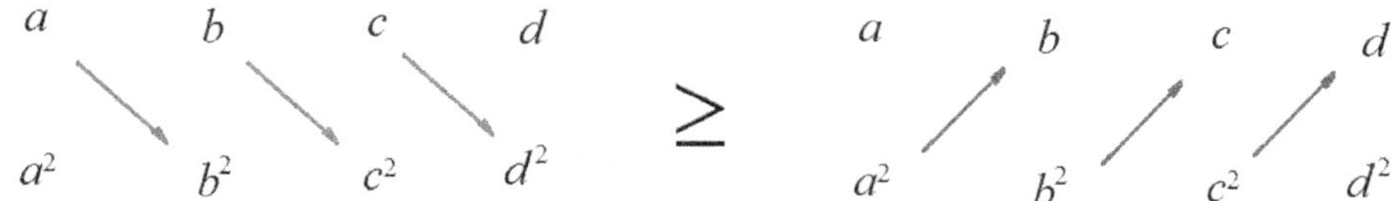

Combining them, we get the following inequalities:

$$ab^2 + bc^2 + cd^2 + da^2 \ge a^2b + b^2c + c^2d + d^2a \quad (1)$$

Method 2:

The inequality is equivalent to

$\Rightarrow \ ab^2 + bc^2 + cd^2 + da^2 - a^2b - b^2c - c^2d - d^2a \ge 0$

$\Rightarrow \ (ab^2 - d^2a) + (bc^2 - a^2b) + (cd^2 - b^2c) + (da^2 - c^2d) \ge 0$

$\Rightarrow \ (d^2 - b^2)(c - a) - (c^2 - a^2)(d - b) \ge 0$

$\Rightarrow \ (d - b)(c - a)[(d - c) + (b - a)] \ge 0$.

The last inequality is certainly true.

Example 3. If $0 \le a \le b \le c \le d$, show that $a^4 + b^4 + c^4 + d^4 \ge ab^3 + bc^3 + cd^3 + da^3$.

Solution:

For the following similarly ordered sequences,

$a, \ b, \ c, \ d$

a^3, b^3, c^3, d^3

By the rearrangement inequality, we have

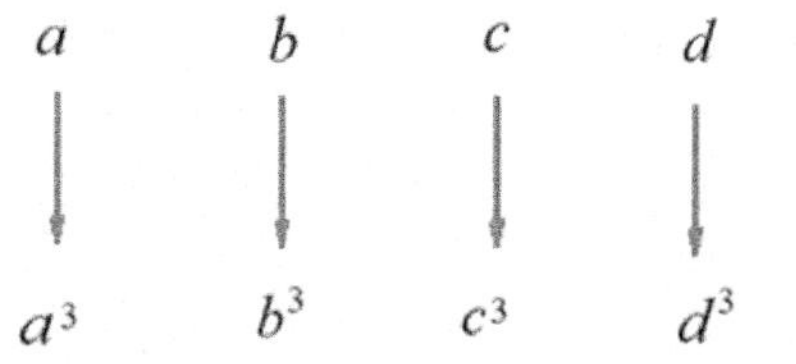

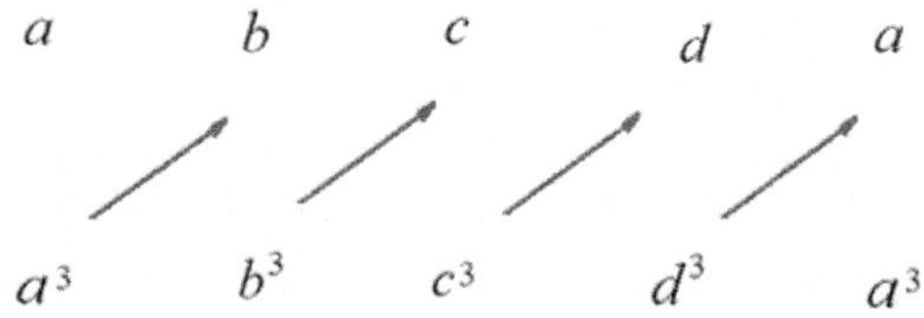

$a^4 + b^4 + c^4 + d^4 \geq a^3b + b^3c + c^3d + d^3a.$

Example 4. If $0 \leq a \leq b \leq c \leq d$, show that $a^5 + b^5 + c^5 + d^5 \geq a^2b^3 + b^2c^3 + c^2d^3 + d^2a^3$.

Solution:

For the following similarly ordered sequences,

$a^2,\ b^2,\ c^2,\ d^2$

a^3, b^3, c^3, d^3

By the rearrangement inequality, we have

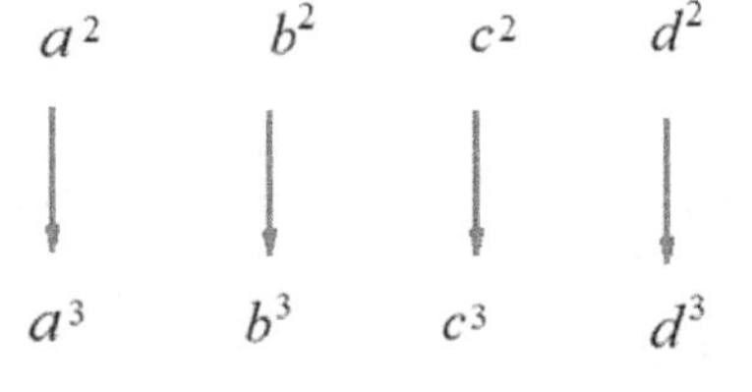

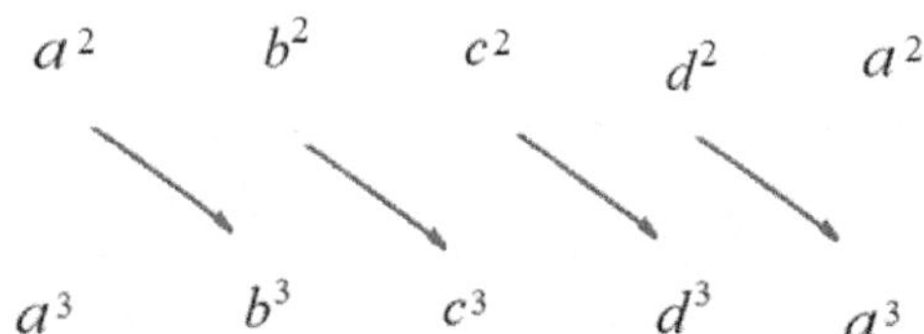

$a^5 + b^5 + c^5 + d^5 \geq a^2b^3 + b^2c^3 + c^2d^3 + d^2a^3.$

Example 5. If $0 \leq a \leq b \leq c \leq d$, show that $a^3b + b^3c + c^3d + d^3a \geq a^3d + b^3c + c^3b + d^3a$.

Solution:

For the following similarly ordered sequences,

a, b, c, d

d^3, c^3, b^3, a^3

by the rearrangement inequality, we have

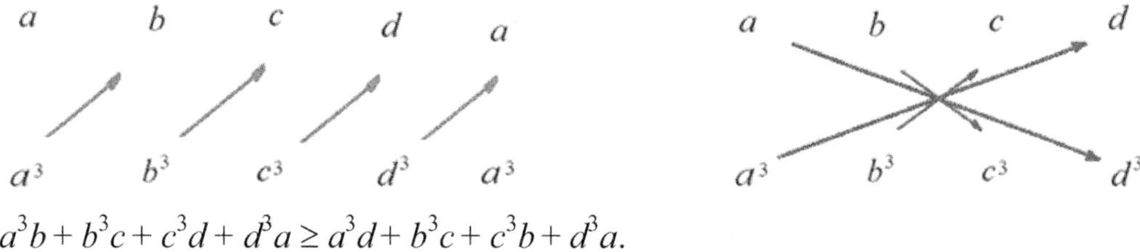

$a^3b + b^3c + c^3d + d^3a \geq a^3d + b^3c + c^3b + d^3a.$

Example 6. For nonnegative numbers a, b, c, d, show that $a^2 + b^2 + c^2 + d^2 \geq ab + bc + cd + da$.

Solution:

For the following similarly ordered sequences,

a, b, c, d

d^3, c^3, b^3, a^3

by the rearrangement inequality, we have

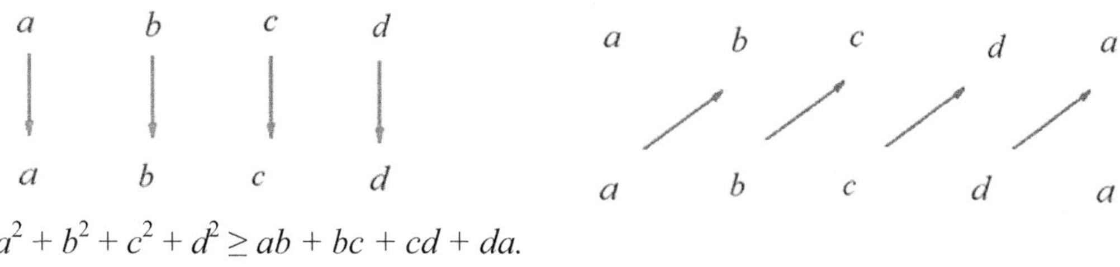

$a^2 + b^2 + c^2 + d^2 \geq ab + bc + cd + da.$

Example 7. Prove that for all positive real numbers $a \leq b \leq c$, $\frac{a^4}{b^2} + \frac{b^4}{a^2} \geq 2ab$.

Solution:

Since $a \leq b$, we know that $\frac{1}{b} \leq \frac{1}{a}$

Then we have the following two similarly ordered sequences:

$a^3, b^3,$

$\frac{a}{b^2}, \frac{b}{a^2}$

By the rearrangement inequality, we have

a^3 b^3 a^3 b^3

$\frac{a}{b^2}$ $\frac{b}{a^2}$ $\frac{a}{b^2}$ $\frac{b}{a^2}$

$\frac{a^4}{b^2} + \frac{b^4}{a^2} \ge a^3 \cdot \frac{b}{a^2} + b^3 \cdot \frac{a}{b^2} = 2ab.$

Example 8. Prove that for all positive real numbers $a \le b \le c$, $\frac{a^3}{b} + \frac{b^3}{c} + \frac{c^3}{a} \ge ab + bc + ca$.

Solution:

Since $a \le b \le c$, we know that $\frac{1}{c} \le \frac{1}{b} \le \frac{1}{a}$

Then we have the following two similarly ordered sequences:

a^3, b^3, c^3.

$\frac{1}{c}, \frac{1}{b}, \frac{1}{a}$

By the rearrangement inequality, we have

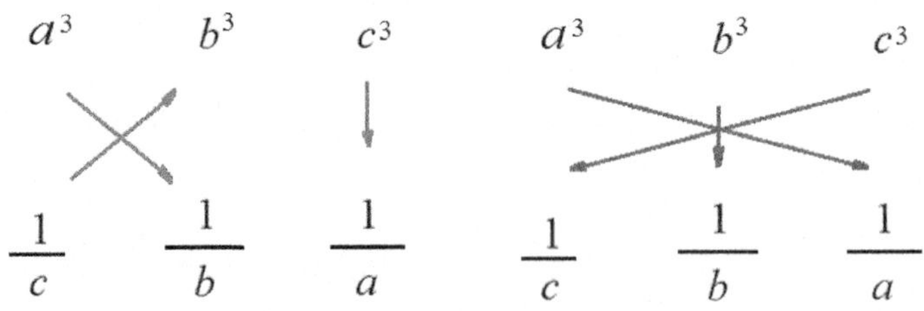

$\frac{a^3}{b} + \frac{b^3}{c} + \frac{c^3}{a} \ge a^3 \cdot \frac{1}{a} + b^3 \cdot \frac{1}{b} + c^3 \cdot \frac{1}{c}$
$= a^2 + b^2 + c^2 \ge ab + bc + ca$.

Method 2:

From AM-GM, we have

$$\frac{a^3}{b}+\frac{b^3}{c}+bc \geq 3\sqrt[3]{\frac{a^3}{b}\cdot\frac{b^3}{c}\cdot bc}=3ab \qquad (1)$$

Similarly,

$$\frac{b^3}{c}+\frac{c^3}{a}+ca \geq 3bc \qquad (2)$$

$$\frac{c^3}{a}+\frac{a^3}{b}+ab \geq 3ca \qquad (3)$$

(1) + (2) + (3):

$$2(\frac{a^3}{b^2}+\frac{b^3}{c^2}+\frac{c^3}{a^2})+ab\ +\ bc\ +\ ca \geq 3(ab+bc+ca)$$

That is $\frac{a^3}{b^2}+\frac{b^3}{c^2}+\frac{c^3}{a^2}\geq ab\ +\ bc\ +ca.$

Equality holds iff $a = b = c$.

Example 9. For $0 < a \leq b \leq c$, show that $a^{2a}b^{2b}c^{2c} \geq a^{b+c}b^{c+a}c^{a+b}$.

Solution:

For the following similarly ordered two sequences,

$a,\quad b,\quad c$

$\log a, \log b, \log c$

We have :

$$a\log a + b\log b + c\log c \geq a\log b + b\log c + c\log a \qquad (1)$$

$$a\log a + b\log b + c\log c \geq b\log a + c\log b + a\log c \qquad (2)$$

(1) + (2):

$$2a\log a + 2b\log b + 2c\log c \geq (b+c)\log a + (c+a)\log b + (a+b)\log c$$

$$\Rightarrow \log a^{2a} + \log b^{2b} + \log c^{2c} \geq \log a^{b+c} + \log b^{c+a} + \log c^{a+b}$$

$$\Rightarrow \log(a^{2a}\cdot b^{2b}\cdot c^{2c}) \geq \log(a^{b+c}\cdot b^{c+a}\cdot c^{a+b})$$

$$\Rightarrow a^{2a}\cdot b^{2b}\cdot c^{2c} \geq a^{b+c}\cdot b^{c+a}\cdot c^{a+b}.$$

Example 10. If $0 \leq a \leq b \leq c$, show that $\frac{a^5}{b^3c^3}+\frac{b^5}{c^3a^3}+\frac{c^5}{a^3b^3} \geq \frac{1}{a}+\frac{1}{b}+\frac{1}{c}.$

Solution:

Since $a \le b \le c$, we have the following two similarly ordered sequences:

$a^3,\ b^3,\ c^3$

$\frac{1}{b^3c^3}, \frac{1}{c^3a^3}, \frac{1}{a^3b^3}$.

By the rearrangement inequality, we have

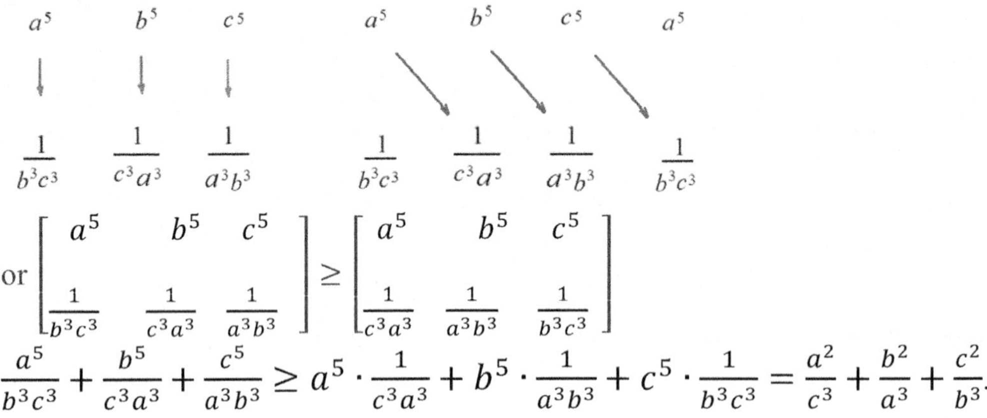

$$\frac{a^5}{b^3c^3} + \frac{b^5}{c^3a^3} + \frac{c^5}{a^3b^3} \ge a^5 \cdot \frac{1}{c^3a^3} + b^5 \cdot \frac{1}{a^3b^3} + c^5 \cdot \frac{1}{b^3c^3} = \frac{a^2}{c^3} + \frac{b^2}{a^3} + \frac{c^2}{b^3}.$$

By the rearrangement inequality again, we have

$$\begin{matrix} a^2 & b^2 & c^2 \\ \downarrow & \times & \\ \frac{1}{c^3} & \frac{1}{b^3} & \frac{1}{a^3} \end{matrix} \qquad \begin{matrix} a^2 & b^2 & c^2 \\ & \times\!\downarrow & \\ \frac{1}{c^3} & \frac{1}{b^3} & \frac{1}{a^3} \end{matrix}$$

or $\begin{bmatrix} a^2 & b^2 & c^2 \\ \frac{1}{c^3} & \frac{1}{a^3} & \frac{1}{b^3} \end{bmatrix} \ge \begin{bmatrix} a^2 & b^2 & c^2 \\ \frac{1}{a^3} & \frac{1}{b^3} & \frac{1}{c^3} \end{bmatrix}$

$$\frac{a^2}{c^3} + \frac{b^2}{a^3} + \frac{c^2}{b^3} \ge a^2 \cdot \frac{1}{a^3} + b^2 \cdot \frac{1}{b^3} + c^2 \cdot \frac{1}{c^3} = \frac{1}{a} + \frac{1}{b} + \frac{1}{c}.$$ QED.

Example 11. Let $0 \le a \le b \le c \le d$. Prove that $\frac{a^3+b^3+c^3}{a+b+c} + \frac{b^3+c^3+d^3}{b+c+d} + \frac{c^3+d^3+a^3}{c+d+a} + \frac{d^3+a^3+b^3}{d+a+b} \ge a^2 + b^2 + c^2 + d^2$.

Solution:

Since $a \le b \le c \le d$, we have $a + b + c \le a + b + d \le a + c + d \le b + c + d$.
Then we have the following two similarly ordered sequences:
$a^3 + b^3 + c^3$, $a^3 + b^3 + d^3$, $a^3 + c^3 + d^3$, $b^3 + c^3 + d^3$,
$\frac{1}{b+c+d}, \frac{1}{c+a+d}, \frac{1}{a+b+d}, \frac{1}{a+b+c}$.

By the rearrangement inequality, we have

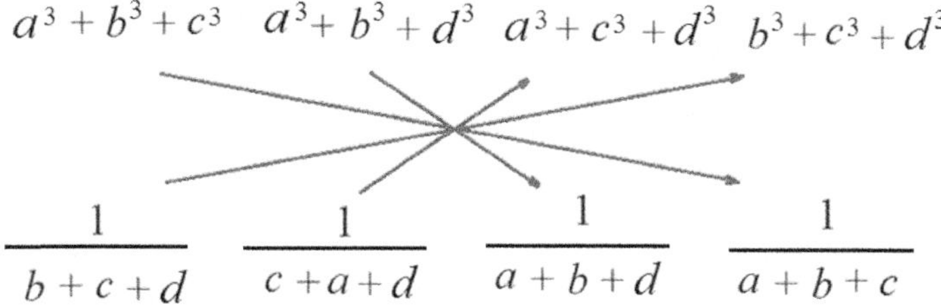

We see that $\frac{a^3+b^3+c^3}{a+b+c} + \frac{b^3+c^3+d^3}{b+c+d} + \frac{c^3+d^3+a^3}{c+d+a} + \frac{d^3+a^3+b^3}{d+a+b}$ is opposite ordered and it is the smallest possible value of any arrangements. We are not able to use the rearrangement inequality directly to solve this problem.

Now we try to prove the following inequality:
$\frac{a^3+b^3+c^3}{a+b+c} \ge \frac{a^2+b^2+c^2}{3}$.

Since the inequality is symmetric, WLOG, we may assume that $a \le b \le c$. Then we know that $a^2 \le b^2 \le c^2$.

Then we have the following two similarly ordered sequences:
a, b, c.
a^2, b^2, c^2.

By the rearrangement inequality, we have

$$\begin{array}{ccc} a & b & c \\ \downarrow & \downarrow & \downarrow \\ a^2 & b^2 & c^2 \end{array} \qquad \begin{array}{cccc} a & b & c & a \\ \searrow & \searrow & \searrow & \\ a^2 & b^2 & c^2 & a^2 \end{array}$$

$$a^3 + b^3 + c^3 \geq ab^2 + bc^2 + ca^2 \qquad (1)$$

$$\begin{array}{ccc} a & b & c \\ \downarrow & \downarrow & \downarrow \\ a^2 & b^2 & c^2 \end{array} \qquad \begin{array}{cccc} a & b & c & a \\ \nearrow & \nearrow & \nearrow & \\ a^2 & b^2 & c^2 & a^2 \end{array}$$

$$a^3 + b^3 + c^3 \geq a^2b + b^2c + c^2a \qquad (2)$$

We certainly have

$$a^3 + b^3 + c^3 \geq a^3 + b^3 + c^3 \qquad (3)$$

(1) + (2) + (3):

$$3(a^3 + b^3 + c^3) \geq (a^3 + ca^2 + ba^2) + (b^3 + cb^2 + ab^2) + c^3 + bc^2 + c^2a)$$

$$= (a + b + b)(a^2 + b^2 + c^2)$$

Or

$$\frac{a^3 + b^3 + c^3}{a + b + c} \geq \frac{a^2 + b^2 + c^2}{3}$$

Similarly,

$$\frac{b^3 + c^3 + d^3}{b + c + d} \geq \frac{b^2 + c^2 + d^2}{3}$$

$$\frac{c^3 + d^3 + a^3}{c + d + a} \geq \frac{c^2 + d^2 + a^2}{3}$$

$$\frac{d^3 + a^3 + b^3}{d + a + b} \geq \frac{d^2 + a^2 + b^2}{3}$$

$$\frac{a^3+b^3+c^3}{a+b+c} + \frac{b^3+c^3+d^3}{b+c+d} + \frac{c^3+d^3+a^3}{c+d+a} + \frac{d^3+a^3+b^3}{d+a+b}$$

$$\geq \frac{a^2+b^2+c^2}{3} + \frac{b^2+c^2+d^2}{3} + \frac{c^2+d^2+a^2}{3} + \frac{d^2+a^2+b^2}{3}$$

$$= a^2 + b^2 + c^2 + d^2.$$

Example 12. If $a \le b \le c \le d$, show that $a^2bc + b^2ad + c^2bd + d^2ac \ge 4abcd$.

Solution:
Since $a \le b \le c \le d$, we have $abc \le abd \le acd \le bcd$.

Then we have the following two similarly ordered sequences:
$a, b, c, d,$
$abc, abd, acd, bcd.$

By the rearrangement inequality, we have

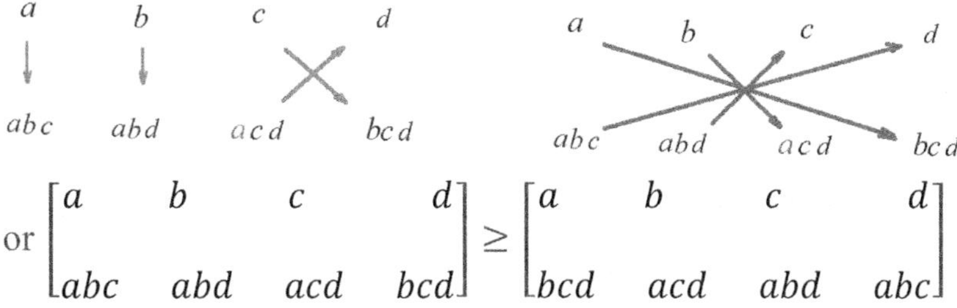

or $\begin{bmatrix} a & b & c & d \\ abc & abd & acd & bcd \end{bmatrix} \ge \begin{bmatrix} a & b & c & d \\ bcd & acd & abd & abc \end{bmatrix}$

That is, $a^2bc + b^2ad + c^2bd + d^2ac \ge 4abcd$.

Example 13. Show that for real positive numbers a, b, c, $\frac{a^2}{b^2} + \frac{b^2}{c^2} + \frac{c^2}{a^2} \ge \frac{a}{b} + \frac{b}{c} + \frac{c}{a}$.

Proof:
Method 1:
The following sequences are similarly arranged.
$a^2, b^2\ c^2$
$\frac{1}{c^2}, \frac{1}{b^2}, \frac{1}{c^2}$

By the rearrangement inequality (**Theorem 3.4**), we have

$$a^2 \quad b^2 \quad c^2 \qquad\qquad a^2 \quad b^2 \quad c^2$$

$$\frac{1}{c^2} \quad \frac{1}{b^2} \quad \frac{1}{a^2} \qquad\qquad \frac{1}{c^2} \quad \frac{1}{b^2} \quad \frac{1}{a^2}$$

$$\frac{a^2}{b^2}+\frac{b^2}{c^2}+\frac{c^2}{a^2}\geq \frac{a^2}{c^2}+\frac{b^2}{a^2}+\frac{c^2}{b^2} \qquad (1)$$

The following triplets are similarly arranged.

$\frac{a}{c}, \frac{c}{b}, \frac{b}{a}$

$\frac{a}{c}, \frac{c}{b}, \frac{b}{a}$

By the rearrangement inequality, we have

$$\frac{a}{c} \quad \frac{c}{b} \quad \frac{b}{a} \qquad\qquad \frac{a}{c} \quad \frac{c}{b} \quad \frac{b}{a} \quad \frac{a}{c}$$

$$\frac{a}{c} \quad \frac{c}{b} \quad \frac{b}{a} \qquad\qquad \frac{a}{c} \quad \frac{c}{b} \quad \frac{b}{a} \quad \frac{a}{c}$$

$$\frac{a^2}{c^2}+\frac{b^2}{a^2}+\frac{c^2}{b^2}\geq \frac{a}{c}\cdot\frac{c}{b}+\frac{c}{b}\cdot\frac{b}{a}+\frac{b}{a}\cdot\frac{a}{c}=\frac{a}{b}+\frac{c}{a}+\frac{b}{c} \qquad (2)$$

Thus we get: $\frac{a^2}{b^2}+\frac{b^2}{c^2}+\frac{c^2}{a^2}\geq \frac{a^2}{c^2}+\frac{b^2}{a^2}+\frac{c^2}{b^2}\geq \frac{a}{b}+\frac{c}{a}+\frac{b}{c}$. QED.

Method 2:

Let $x=\frac{a}{b}, y=\frac{b}{c}, z=\frac{c}{a}$. We have $xyz = 1$.

The given inequality becomes

$x^2+y^2+z^2 \geq x+y+z$

From AM-GM, we have

$$\sqrt{\frac{x^2+y^2+z^2}{3}} \geq \frac{x+y+z}{3}$$

i,e, $x^2 + y^2 + z^2 \geq \frac{(x+y+z)^2}{3} \geq \frac{3\sqrt[3]{xyz}(x+y+z)}{3} = x + y + z$.

Method 3: [1] provide the following solution:

Clear the denominators. You will get

$x^4z^2 + y^4x^2 + z^4y^2 \geq x^3yz^2 + x^2y^3z + xy^2z^3$

Now, suppose that $x \geq y \geq z$. Then we transform as follows:

$x^3z^2(x - y) + x^2y^3(y - z) + y^2z^3(z - x) \geq 0$.

Here the first two parentheses are ≥ 0, but the third is not positive. In this case one usually writes $z - x = z - y + y - x$ and collects terms:

$x^3z^2(x - y) + x^2y^3(y - z) - y^2z^3(x - y) - y^2z^3(y - z) \geq 0 \Rightarrow$

$z^2(x^3 - y^2z)(x - y) + y^2(x^2y - z^3)(y - z) \geq 0$

The last inequality is obviously correct.

Example 14. Let *a, b, c* be positive real numbers. Prove that $\frac{a^2}{b} + \frac{b^2}{c} + \frac{c^2}{a}$ $\geq \frac{a^2}{c} + \frac{b^2}{a} + \frac{c^2}{b}$.

Proof:

For the following similarly sorted sequences,

a^2, b^2, c^2.

$\frac{1}{c}, \frac{1}{b}, \frac{1}{a}$

by the rearrangement inequality (**Theorem 3.5**), we have

$$\begin{array}{cccccc} a^2 & b^2 & c^2 & a^2 & b^2 & c^2 \\ \frac{1}{c} & \frac{1}{b} & \frac{1}{a} & \frac{1}{c} & \frac{1}{b} & \frac{1}{a} \end{array}$$

$$\frac{a^2}{b} + \frac{b^2}{c} + \frac{c^2}{a} \geq \frac{a^2}{c} + \frac{b^2}{a} + \frac{c^2}{b}.$$

CHAPTER 3. PROBLEMS

Problem 1. If $0 \le a \le b \le c$, show that $ab^3 + bc^3 + ca^3 \ge a^3 b + b^3 c + c^3 a$.

Problem 2. If $0 \le a \le b \le c \le d$, show that $ab^3 + bc^3 + cd^3 + da^3 \ge a^3 b + b^3 c + c^3 d + d^3 a$.

Problem 3. If $0 \le a \le b \le c \le d$, show that $a^4 + b^4 + c^4 + d^4 \ge ab^3 + bc^3 + cd^3 + da^3$.

Problem 4. If $0 \le a \le b \le c \le d$, show that $a^5 + b^5 + c^5 + d^5 \ge a^3 b^2 + b^3 c^2 + c^3 d^2 + d^3 a^2$.

Problem 5. If n is a positive integer and $0 \le a \le b \le c \le d$, show that

$$ab^5 + bc^5 + cd^5 + da^5 \ge a^5 b + b^5 c + c^5 d + d^5 a.$$

Problem 6. For nonnegative numbers a, b, c, d, show that $a^2 + b^2 + c^2 + d^2 \ge ac + bc + cd + da$.

Problem 7. Prove that for all positive real numbers $a \le b \le c$, $\frac{a^2 b}{c} + \frac{b^2 c}{a} + \frac{c^2 a}{b} \ge ab + bc + ca$.

Problem 8. Prove that for all positive real numbers a, b, c $(a \le b \le c)$, we have $\frac{a^5}{b^3} + \frac{b^5}{c^3} + \frac{c^5}{a^3} \ge a^2 + b^2 + c^2$.

Problem 9. If $1 < a \le b \le c$, then $a^a b^b c^c \ge a^c b^a c^b \ge a^b b^c c^a$.

Problem 10. If $0 \le a \le b \le c$, show that $\frac{a^{12}}{bc} + \frac{b^{12}}{ca} + \frac{c^{12}}{ab} \ge a^{10} + b^{10} + c^{10}$.

Problem 11. Let $0 \le a \le b \le c \le d$. Prove that $\frac{a^3+b^3+c^3}{b+c+d} + \frac{a^3+b^3+d^3}{c+a+d} + \frac{a^3+c^3+d^3}{a+b+d} + \frac{b^3+c^3+d^3}{a+b+c} \ge a^2 + b^2 + c^2 + d^2$.

Problem 12. If $a \le b \le c \le d$, show that $a^2bd + b^2ac + c^2ad + d^2bc \ge 4abcd$.

Problem 13. If a and b are positive real numbers such that $a^4 + b^4 = 1$. Show that $\sqrt[3]{a+b} \ge \sqrt{a^2+b^2}$.

Problem 14. Let a, b, c be positive real numbers. Prove that $\frac{a^3}{b^2} + \frac{b^3}{c^2} + \frac{c^3}{a^2} \ge \frac{a^3}{c^2} + \frac{b^3}{a^2} + \frac{c^3}{b^2}$.

CHAPTER 3. SOLUTIONS

Problem 1. Solution:

Method 1:

We have the following two similarly ordered sequences.

$a, \ b, c$

a^3, b^3, c^3

By the rearrangement inequality, we have

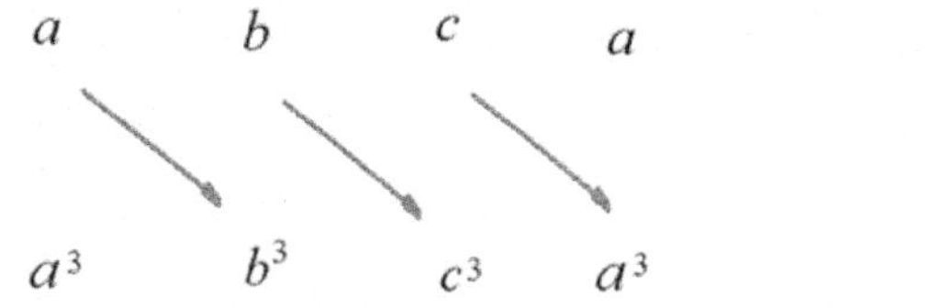

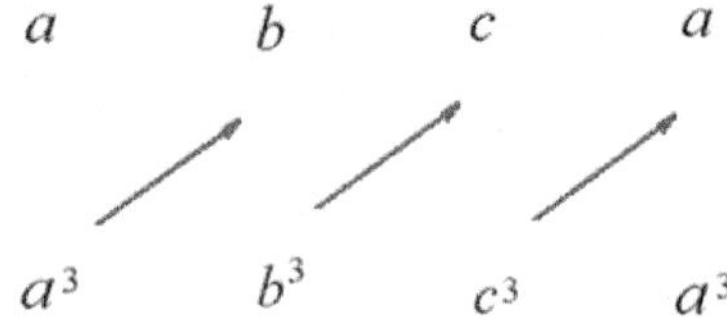

$ab^3 + bc^3 + ca^3 \geq a^3 b + b^3c + c^3a.$

Method 2:

$ab^3 + bc^3 + ca^3 \geq a^3 b + b^3c + c^3a \quad \Leftrightarrow ab^3 + bc^3 + ca^3 - (a^3 b + b^3c + c^3a) \geq 0$

$ab^3 + bc^3 + ca^3 - (a^3 b + b^3c + c^3a)$

$= (ab^3 - a^3 b) + (bc^3 - c^3a) + (ca^3 - b^3c)$

$= ab(b^2 - a^2) + c^3 (b - a) + c(a^3 - b^3)$

$= (b - a)[c (c - b)(c + b) + a(b + a)(b - c)]$

$= (b - a)(c - b) [c (c + b) - a(b + a)]$

$= (b - a)(c - b)(c^2 + cb - ab - a^2)$

$= (b - a)(c - b)(c - a)(c + b + a) \geq 0$. QED.

Problem 2. Solution:

For the following similarly ordered sequences,

a, b, c, d

d^3, c^3, b^3, a^3

by the rearrangement inequality, we have

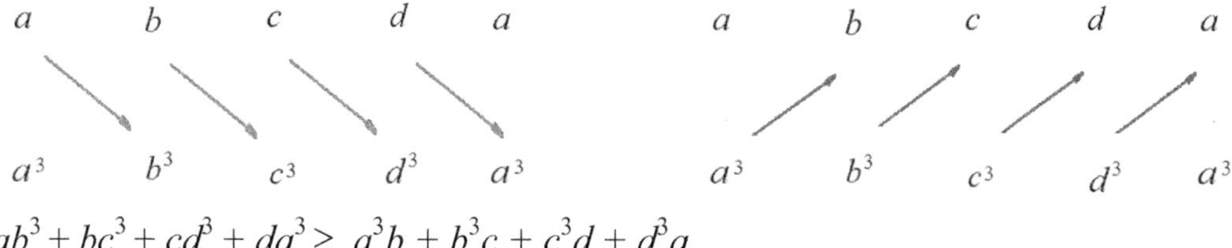

$ab^3 + bc^3 + cd^3 + da^3 \geq a^3b + b^3c + c^3d + d^3a.$

Problem 3. Solution:

For the following similarly ordered sequences,

$a,\ b,\ c,\ d$

a^3, b^3, c^3, d^3

By the rearrangement inequality, we have

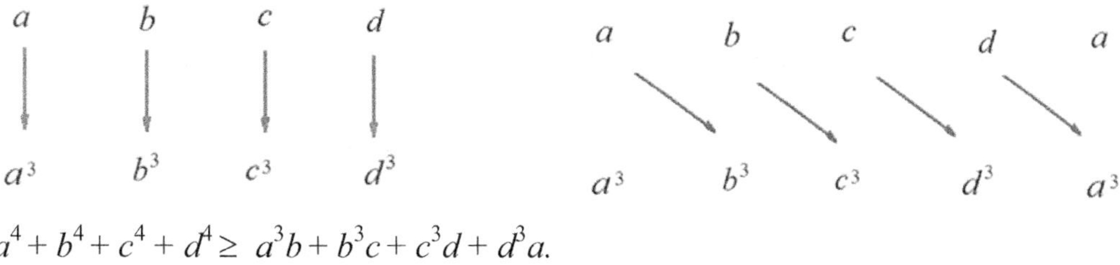

$a^4 + b^4 + c^4 + d^4 \geq a^3b + b^3c + c^3d + d^3a.$

Problem 4. Solution:

For the following similarly ordered sequences,

$a^2,\ b^2,\ c^2,\ d^2$

a^3, b^3, c^3, d^3

By the rearrangement inequality, we have

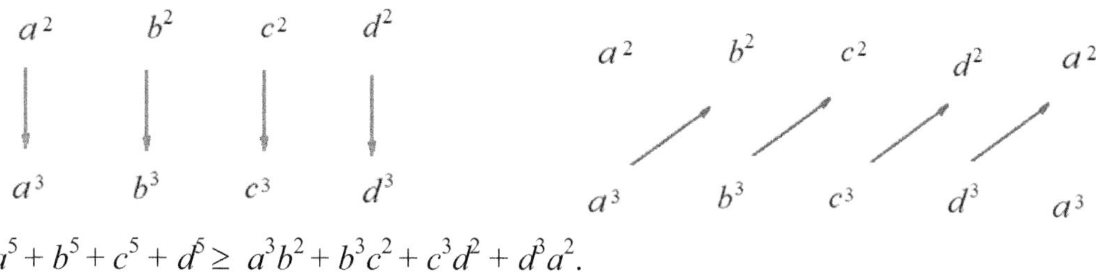

$a^5 + b^5 + c^5 + d^5 \geq a^3b^2 + b^3c^2 + c^3d^2 + d^3a^2.$

Problem 5. Proof:

Method 1:
For the following similarly ordered sequences,
a, b, c, d
a^5, b^5, c^5, d^5
by the rearrangement inequality, we have

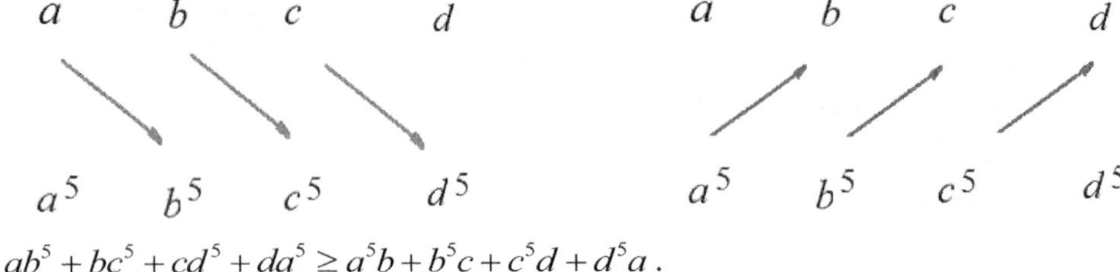

$ab^5 + bc^5 + cd^5 + da^5 \geq a^5b + b^5c + c^5d + d^5a$.

Method 2:
The inequality is equivalent to $ab^5 + bc^5 + cd^5 + da^5 \geq a^5b + b^5c + c^5d + d^5a$.
$\Leftrightarrow$
$ab^5 + bc^5 + cd^5 + da^5 - (a^5b + b^5c + c^5d + d^5a) \geq 0$.
$\Leftrightarrow (d^5 - b^5)(c - a) - (c^5 - d^5)(d - b) \geq 0$
$\Leftrightarrow (d - b)(c - a)[(d^4 + d^3b + d^2b^2 + db^3 + b^4) - (c^4 + c^3a + c^2a^2 + ca^3 + a^4)] \geq 0.$
The last inequality is certainly true.

Problem 6. Solution:
For the following similarly ordered sequences,
a, b, c, d
a, b, c, d
by the rearrangement inequality, we have

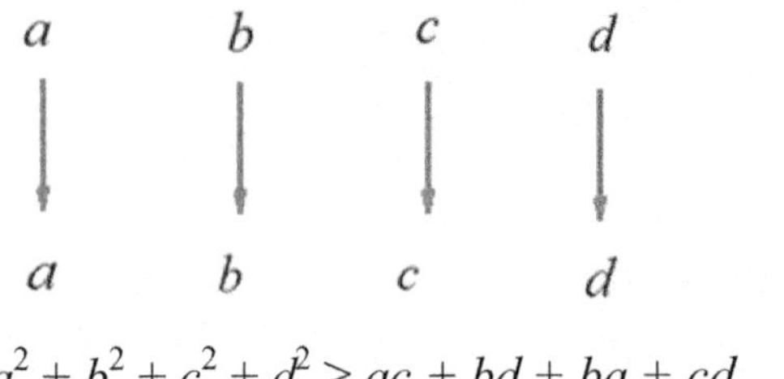

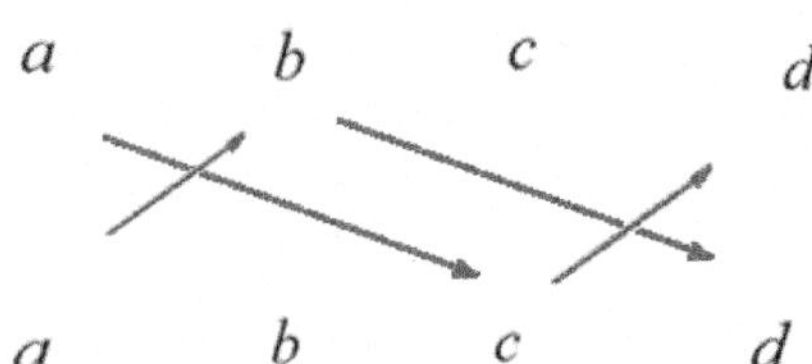

$a^2 + b^2 + c^2 + d^2 \geq ac + bd + ba + cd.$

Problem 7. Solution:

Since $a \le b \le c$, we know that $ab \le ac \le bc$,

$$\frac{ab}{c} \le \frac{ac}{b} \le \frac{bc}{a}$$

Then we have the following two similarly ordered sequences:

$a, b, c,$

$\frac{ab}{c}, \frac{ac}{b}, \frac{bc}{a}.$

By the rearrangement inequality, we have

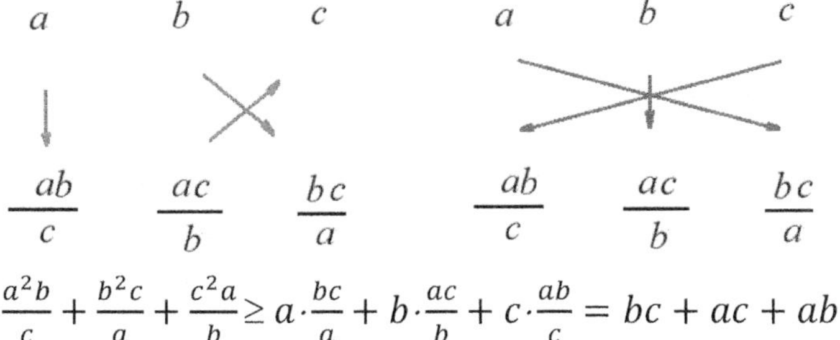

$$\frac{a^2b}{c} + \frac{b^2c}{a} + \frac{c^2a}{b} \ge a\cdot\frac{bc}{a} + b\cdot\frac{ac}{b} + c\cdot\frac{ab}{c} = bc + ac + ab\ .$$

Problem 8. Solution:

Method 1:

Since $a \le b \le c$, we have $a^5 \le b^5 \le c^5$, and $\frac{1}{c^3} \le \frac{1}{b^3} \le \frac{1}{a^3}$

Then we have the following two similarly ordered sequences:

$a^5, b^5, c^5.$

$\frac{1}{c^3}, \frac{1}{b^3}, \frac{1}{a^3}$

By the rearrangement inequality, we have

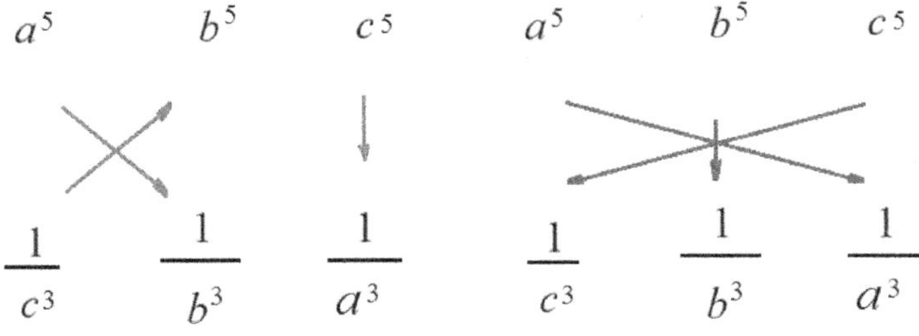

$$\frac{a^5}{b^3}+\frac{b^5}{c^3}+\frac{c^5}{a^3} \geq a^5 \cdot \frac{1}{a^3}+b^5 \cdot \frac{1}{b^3}+c^5 \cdot \frac{1}{c^3}=a^2+b^2+c^2.$$

Method 2:
From AM-GM, we have

$$2\frac{a^5}{b^3}+3b^2=\frac{a^5}{b^3}+\frac{a^5}{b^3}+b^2+b^2+b^2 \geq 5\sqrt[5]{\frac{a^5}{b^3}\cdot\frac{a^5}{b^3}\cdot b^2 \cdot b^2 \cdot b^2}=5a^2 \qquad (1)$$

Similarly,

$$2\frac{b^5}{c^3}+3c^2 \geq 5b^2 \qquad (2)$$

$$2\frac{b^5}{c^3}+3c^2 \geq 5b^2 \qquad (3)$$

(1) + (2) + (3):

$$2\left(\frac{a^5}{b^3}+\frac{b^5}{c^3}+\frac{c^5}{a^3}\right)+3(a^2+b^2+c^2) \geq 5(a^2+b^2+c^2).$$

That is $\frac{a^5}{b^3}+\frac{b^5}{c^3}+\frac{c^5}{a^3} \geq a^2+b^2+c^2$.
Equality holds iff $a = b = c$.

Problem 9. Solution:
For the following similarly ordered two sequences,

$a, \quad b, \quad c$
$\log a, \log b, \log c$

we have the following inequality holds

$$a\log a+b\log b+c\log c \geq a\log b+b\log c+c\log a \geq b\log a+c\log b+a\log c \qquad (1)$$

$$\Rightarrow \log(a^a \cdot b^b \cdot c^c) \geq \log(b^a \cdot c^b \cdot a^c) \geq \log(a^b \cdot b^c \cdot c^a)$$

$$\Rightarrow a^a b^b c^c \geq a^c b^a c^b \geq a^b b^c c^a.$$

Problem 10. Solution:
Since $a \leq b \leq c$, we have the following two similarly ordered sequences:

$a^{12}, \ b^{12}, \ c^{12}$
$\frac{1}{bc}, \frac{1}{ca}, \frac{1}{ab}.$

By the rearrangement inequality, we have

$$\begin{matrix} a^{12} & b^{12} & c^{12} \\ \downarrow & \downarrow & \downarrow \\ \frac{1}{bc} & \frac{1}{ac} & \frac{1}{ab} \end{matrix} \qquad \begin{matrix} a^{12} & b^{12} & c^{12} & a^{12} \\ \searrow & \searrow & \searrow & \\ \frac{1}{bc} & \frac{1}{ac} & \frac{1}{ab} & \frac{1}{bc} \end{matrix}$$

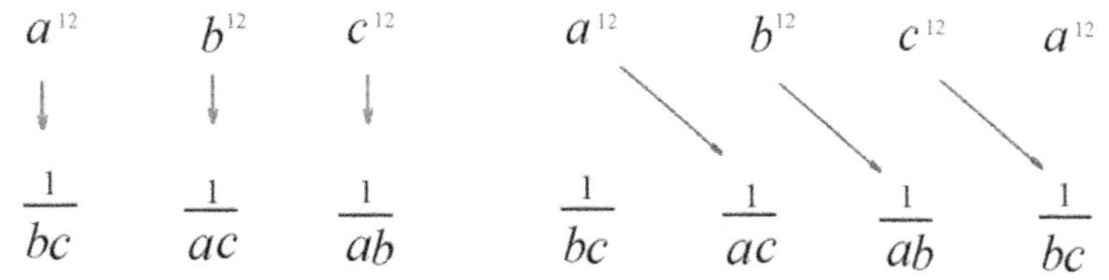

or $\begin{bmatrix} a^{12} & b^{12} & c^{12} \\ \frac{1}{bc} & \frac{1}{ca} & \frac{1}{ab} \end{bmatrix} \ge \begin{bmatrix} a^{12} & b^{12} & c^{12} \\ \frac{1}{ab} & \frac{1}{bc} & \frac{1}{ac} \end{bmatrix}$

$$\frac{a^{12}}{bc} + \frac{b^{12}}{ca} + \frac{c^{12}}{ab} \ge a^{12} \cdot \frac{1}{ab} + b^{12} \cdot \frac{1}{bc} + c^{12} \cdot \frac{1}{ac} = \frac{a^{11}}{b} + \frac{b^{11}}{c} + \frac{c^{11}}{a}.$$

By the rearrangement inequality again, we have

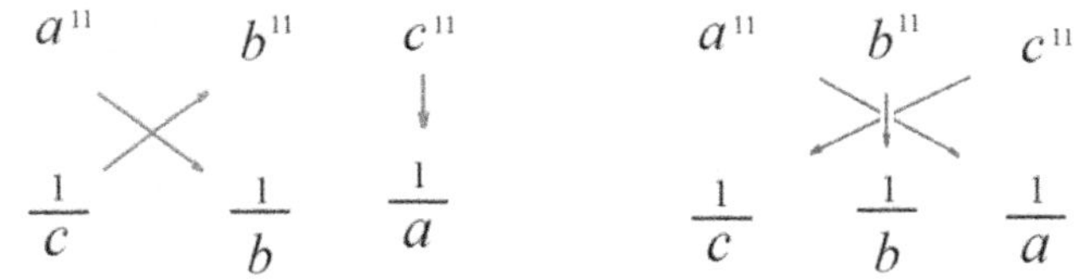

$$\begin{matrix} a^{11} & b^{11} & c^{11} \\ \times & & \downarrow \\ \frac{1}{c} & \frac{1}{b} & \frac{1}{a} \end{matrix} \qquad \begin{matrix} a^{11} & b^{11} & c^{11} \\ & \times & \\ \frac{1}{c} & \frac{1}{b} & \frac{1}{a} \end{matrix}$$

or $\begin{bmatrix} a^{11} & b^{11} & c^{11} \\ \frac{1}{b} & \frac{1}{c} & \frac{1}{a} \end{bmatrix} \ge \begin{bmatrix} a^{11} & b^{11} & c^{11} \\ \frac{1}{a} & \frac{1}{b} & \frac{1}{c} \end{bmatrix}$

$$\frac{a^{11}}{b} + \frac{b^{11}}{c} + \frac{c^{11}}{a} \ge a^{11} \cdot \frac{1}{a} + b^{11} \cdot \frac{1}{b} + c^{11} \cdot \frac{1}{c} = a^{10} + b^{10} + c^{10}.$$

Problem 11. Solution:

Since $a \le b \le c \le d$, we have $a + b + c \le a + b + d \le a + c + d \le b + c + d$.
Then we have the following two similarly ordered sequences:
$a^3 + b^3 + c^3, a^3 + b^3 + d^3, a^3 + c^3 + d^3, b^3 + c^3 + d^3$,
$\frac{1}{b+c+d}, \frac{1}{c+a+d}, \frac{1}{a+b+d}, \frac{1}{a+b+c}$.

By the rearrangement inequality, we have

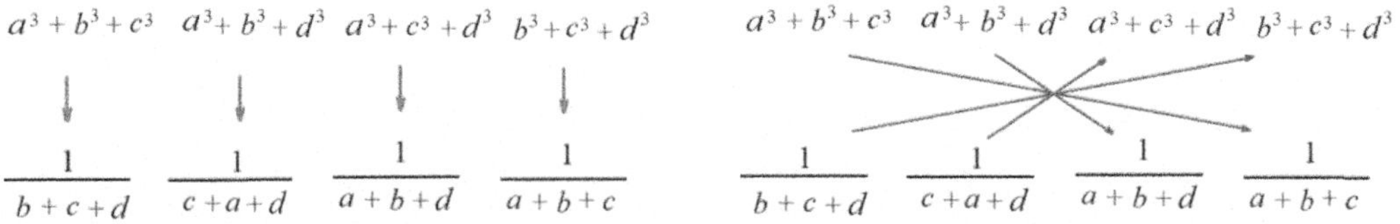

$$\begin{matrix} a^3+b^3+c^3 & a^3+b^3+d^3 & a^3+c^3+d^3 & b^3+c^3+d^3 \\ \downarrow & \downarrow & \downarrow & \downarrow \\ \frac{1}{b+c+d} & \frac{1}{c+a+d} & \frac{1}{a+b+d} & \frac{1}{a+b+c} \end{matrix} \qquad \begin{matrix} a^3+b^3+c^3 & a^3+b^3+d^3 & a^3+c^3+d^3 & b^3+c^3+d^3 \\ \frac{1}{b+c+d} & \frac{1}{c+a+d} & \frac{1}{a+b+d} & \frac{1}{a+b+c} \end{matrix}$$

$$\frac{a^3+b^3+c^3}{b+c+d}+\frac{a^3+b^3+d^3}{a+c+d}+\frac{a^3+c^3+d^3}{a+b+d}+\frac{b^3+c^3+d^3}{a+b+c}$$
$$\geq \frac{a^3+b^3+c^3}{a+b+c}+\frac{b^3+c^3+d^3}{b+c+d}+\frac{c^3+d^3+a^3}{c+d+a}+\frac{d^3+a^3+b^3}{d+a+b}.$$

We know that $\frac{a^3+b^3+c^3}{a+b+c}+\frac{b^3+c^3+d^3}{b+c+d}+\frac{c^3+d^3+a^3}{c+d+a}+\frac{d^3+a^3+b^3}{d+a+b}\geq a^2+b^2+c^2+d^2$.

Thus $\frac{a^3+b^3+c^3}{b+c+d}+\frac{a^3+b^3+d^3}{c+a+d}+\frac{a^3+c^3+d^3}{a+b+d}+\frac{b^3+c^3+d^3}{a+b+c}\geq a^2+b^2+c^2+d^2$.

Problem 12. Solution:

Since $a \leq b \leq c \leq d$, we have $abc \leq abd \leq acd \leq bcd$.

Then we have the following two similarly ordered sequences:

$a, b, c, d,$

$abc, abd, acd, bcd.$

By the rearrangement inequality, we have

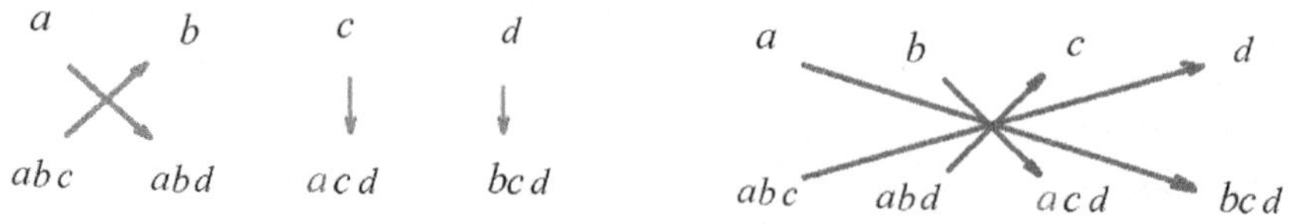

$$\begin{matrix} a & b & c & d \\ & \times & \downarrow & \downarrow \\ abc & abd & acd & bcd \end{matrix} \qquad \begin{matrix} a & b & c & d \\ abc & abd & acd & bcd \end{matrix}$$

or $\begin{bmatrix} a & b & c & d \\ abd & abc & acd & bcd \end{bmatrix} \geq \begin{bmatrix} a & b & c & d \\ bcd & acd & abd & abc \end{bmatrix}$

That is, $a^2bd+b^2ac+c^2ad+d^2bc \geq 4abcd$.

Problem 13. Solution:
Method 1:

The given inequality is equivalent to

$(a+b)^2 \geq (a^2+b^2)^3 \quad \Leftrightarrow a^2+b^2+2ab \geq (a^2+b^2)^2(a^2+b^2)$

$\Leftrightarrow a^2+b^2+2ab \geq (a^4+b^4+2a^2b^2)(a^2+b^2)$

$\Leftrightarrow a^2+b^2+2ab \geq (1+2a^2b^2)(a^2+b^2)$

$\Leftrightarrow a^2+b^2+2ab \geq (a^2+b^2)+2a^2b^2(a^2+b^2)$

$\Leftrightarrow 2ab \geq +2a^2b^2(a^2+b^2)$

$\Leftrightarrow 1 \geq +ab(a^2+b^2)$ or

$a^3b+ab^3 \leq 1.$
By the rearrangement inequality, we have

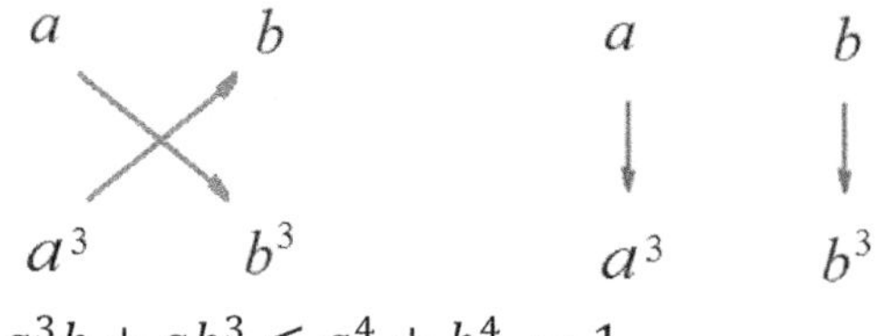

$a^3b+ab^3 \leq a^4+b^4 \;= 1.$

Method 2:
The original inequality can be written as $(a+b)^2 \geq (a^2+b^2)^3$
$\Leftrightarrow (a+b)^2 \geq (a^2+b^2)^2(a^2+b^2)$
$\Leftrightarrow a^2+b^2+2ab \geq (a^4+b^4+2a^2b^2)(a^2+b^2)$
$\Leftrightarrow 2ab \geq (2a^2b^2)(a^2+b^2)$
$\Leftrightarrow a^3b+ab^3 \leq 1.$

By AM-GM,
$a^3b+ab^3 = a\cdot a\cdot a\cdot b + a\cdot b\cdot b\cdot b$
$\leq \frac{1}{4}(a^4+a^4+a^4+b^4) + \frac{1}{4}(a^4+b^4+b^4+b^4)$
$= a^4+b^4 = 1.$

Problem 14. Proof:

The expression is a not symmetric function of *a, b,* and *c*. However, we have the following similarly ordered sequences:

a^3, b^3, c^3.

$\frac{1}{c^2}, \frac{1}{b^2}, \frac{1}{a^2}$

By the rearrangement inequality (**Theorem 3.6**), we have

$$\begin{array}{ccc} a^3 & b^3 & c^3 \\ & \times & \downarrow \\ \frac{1}{c^2} & \frac{1}{b^2} & \frac{1}{a^2} \end{array} \qquad \begin{array}{ccc} a^3 & b^3 & c^3 \\ \downarrow & & \times \\ \frac{1}{c^2} & \frac{1}{b^2} & \frac{1}{a^2} \end{array}$$

$$\frac{a^3}{b^2} + \frac{b^3}{c^2} + \frac{c^3}{a^2} \ge a^3 \cdot \frac{1}{c^2} + b^3 \cdot \frac{1}{a^2} + c^3 \cdot \frac{1}{b^2} = \frac{a^3}{c^2} + \frac{b^3}{a^2} + \frac{c^3}{b^2}.$$ QED.

Chapter 4. Solving Symmetric Inequalities

1. Symmetric Functions

$f(x, y)$ is called a symmetric function if it satisfies $f(x, y) = f(y, x)$.

$f(x, y, z)$ is called symmetrical if it satisfies

$f(x, y, z) = f(x, z, y) = f(y, x, z) = f(y, z, x) = f(z, x, y) = f(z, y, x)$.

$f(a_1, a_2, \ldots a_n)$ is a symmetric expression in $a_1, a_2, \ldots a_n$ if, for any permutation $a'_1, a'_2, \ldots a'_n$, we have $f(a_1, a_2, \ldots a_n) = f(a'_1, a'_2, \ldots a'_n)$.

An easy way to test an expression is symmetric or not is to just switch any two of the variables. If the expression doesn't change, the answer is yes. Otherwise, it is no.

Since f is symmetric, we may assume, without loss of generality, that $a_1 \le a_2 \le \ldots \le a_n$ (or $a_1 \ge a_2 \ge \ldots \ge a_n$). The reason we can do so is because f remains invariant under any permutation of the a_i's. This assumption is quite useful sometimes.

2. Examples of symmetric functions:

$x_1^2 + x_2^2$,

$x_1^3 + x_2^3$,

$x_1^2 + x_2^2 + x_1x_2$,

$x_1^2x_2^2 + x_1^3x_2^3$,

$\frac{1}{x_1} + \frac{1}{x_2}$, $\frac{1}{x_1^2} + \frac{1}{x_2^2}$,

$\frac{1}{x_1^3} + \frac{1}{x_2^3}$.

$a^2 + b^2 + c^2$

$a^2b + a^2c + b^2c + b^2a + c^2a + c^2b$.

$a^2bc + a^2cb + b^2ac + b^2ca + c^2ab + c^2ba.$
$xy + yz + zx$

Any constant function (degree 0 polynomial) is symmetric.
The sum of $x_1 + x_2 + ... + x_n$ is symmetric.
The sum of $x^2_1 + x^2_2 + ... + x^2_n$ is symmetric.
The sum of $x^k_1 + x^k_2 + ... + x^k_n$ is symmetric.

The sum $\sum_{i \le j} x_i x_j$ of all products, including the squares, is symmetric.
The sum $\sum_{i<j} x_i x_j$ of all products, excluding the squares, is symmetric.

Example 1. Is the expression $\frac{a}{b} + \frac{b}{c} + \frac{c}{a}$ symmetric?

Solution: No.
Method :
If we change a for b, we have $\frac{b}{a} + \frac{a}{c} + \frac{c}{b}$ which is different from the given expression. So this expression is not symmetric.

Method 2:
If we switch a and b in the term $\frac{a}{b}$, it becomes $\frac{b}{a}$. We see the term $\frac{b}{c}$ but not $\frac{b}{a}$. So this expression is not symmetric.

Example 2. Is the expression symmetric?
$\frac{a^2+c^2}{b} + \frac{b^2+a^2}{c} + \frac{c^2+a^2}{a}$

Solution: No.
Method 1:
We do the following replacements $a \Leftrightarrow b$, and we get
$\frac{b^2+a^2}{c} + \frac{c^2+b^2}{a} + \frac{a^2+b^2}{b}.$
We see that the new expression is different from the given one. So it is not symmetric.

Method 2:

If we switch a and b in the term $\frac{a^2+c^2}{b}$, it becomes $\frac{b^2+a^2}{c}$. The expression does not match any of the two terms left. So this expression is not symmetric.

Example 3. Is the expression symmetric?

$$\frac{a}{b+c}+\frac{b}{c+a}+\frac{c}{c+b}$$

Solution: Yes.

Method 1:

We do the following replacements $a \Leftrightarrow b$, and we get

$$\frac{b}{a+c}+\frac{a}{c+b}+\frac{c}{c+a}$$

We see that the new expression is the same as the given one. So it is symmetric..

Method 2:

If we switch a and b in the term $\frac{a}{b+c}$, it becomes $\frac{b}{a+c}$. The expression does match the second term ($\frac{b}{c+a}$). So this expression is symmetric.

Example 4. Show that when a, b and c are positive real numbers,

$$(a+b+c)\times(\frac{1}{a}+\frac{1}{b}+\frac{1}{c})\geq 3^2.$$

Solution:

The given inequality is equivalent to the following inequality:

$$\frac{a+b+c}{a}+\frac{a+b+c}{b}+\frac{a+b+c}{c}\geq 9 \text{ or}$$

$$1+\frac{b+c}{a}+1+\frac{a+c}{b}+1+\frac{a+b}{c}\geq 9 \text{ or } \frac{b+c}{a}+\frac{a+c}{b}+\frac{a+b}{c}\geq 6.$$

Since the inequality is symmetric, WLOG, we may assume that $a\leq b\leq c$, $a+b\leq a+c\leq b+c$, and $\frac{1}{c}\leq\frac{1}{b}\leq\frac{1}{a}$

For the following similarly ordered sequences,

$a+b, a+c, b+c$
$\frac{1}{c}, \frac{1}{b}, \frac{1}{a}$

by the rearrangement inequality, we have

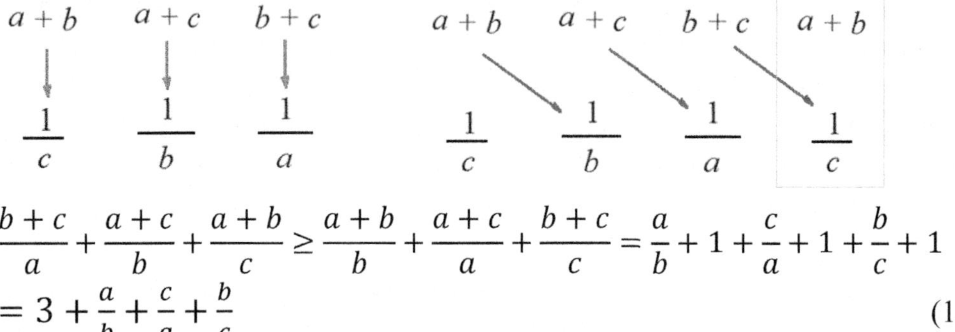

$$\frac{b+c}{a}+\frac{a+c}{b}+\frac{a+b}{c} \geq \frac{a+b}{b}+\frac{a+c}{a}+\frac{b+c}{c}=\frac{a}{b}+1+\frac{c}{a}+1+\frac{b}{c}+1$$
$$= 3+\frac{a}{b}+\frac{c}{a}+\frac{b}{c} \qquad (1)$$

For the following similarly ordered sequences,
a, b, c
$\frac{1}{c}, \frac{1}{b}, \frac{1}{a}$
by the rearrangement inequality, we have

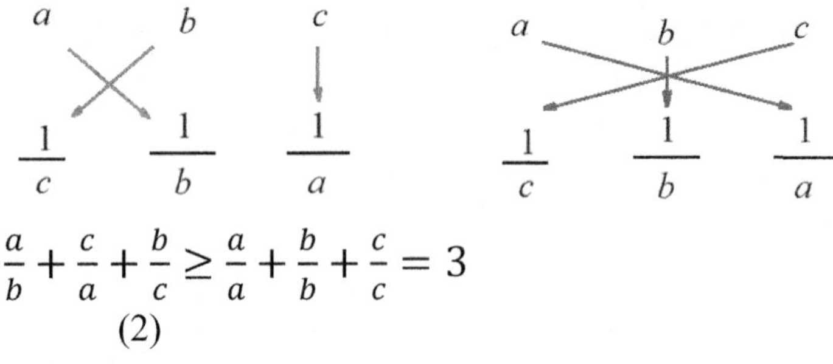

$$\frac{a}{b}+\frac{c}{a}+\frac{b}{c} \geq \frac{a}{a}+\frac{b}{b}+\frac{c}{c}=3$$
(2)

Substituting (2) into (1):
$$\frac{b+c}{a}+\frac{a+c}{b}+\frac{a+b}{c} \geq 3+3=6.$$

Example 5. For all positive numbers a, b and c, prove the inequality

$$\frac{a^2b^2+c^2b^2+c^2a^2}{a+b+c} \geq abc\ .$$

Solution:

The given inequality is equivalent to

$$\frac{a^2b^2+c^2b^2+c^2a^2}{abc} \geq a+b+c, \text{ or}$$

$$\frac{ab}{c}+\frac{ac}{b}+\frac{bc}{a} \geq a+b+c.$$

Since the expression is symmetric, WLOG, we can assume that $a \leq b \leq c$, we know that $ab \leq ac \leq bc$,

$$\frac{1}{c} \leq \frac{b}{b} \leq \frac{1}{a}$$

Then we have the following two similarly ordered sequences:

$ab, ca, bc,$

$\frac{1}{c}, \frac{1}{b}, \frac{1}{a}.$

By the rearrangement inequality, we have

$$\begin{array}{ccc} ab & ac & bc \\ \downarrow & \downarrow & \downarrow \\ \frac{1}{c} & \frac{1}{b} & \frac{1}{a} \end{array} \qquad \begin{array}{cccc} ab & ac & bc & ab \\ \nearrow & \nearrow & \nearrow & \\ \frac{1}{c} & \frac{1}{b} & \frac{1}{a} & \frac{1}{c} \end{array}$$

$$\frac{ab}{c}+\frac{ac}{b}+\frac{bc}{a} \geq ac\cdot\frac{1}{c}+bc\cdot\frac{1}{b}+ab\cdot\frac{1}{a} = a+c+b\ .$$

$$\frac{ab}{c}+\frac{bc}{a}+\frac{ca}{b} \geq a+b+c\ .$$

That is $\frac{a^2b^2+c^2b^2+c^2a^2}{a+b+c} \geq abc$.

Example 6. (Nesbitt's Inequality) Show for positive numbers a, b, c,

$$\frac{a}{b+c}+\frac{b}{c+a}+\frac{c}{a+b}\geq\frac{3}{2}.$$

Solution:

The expression is a symmetric function. WLOG, we let $a \leq b \leq c$.
For the following similarly ordered two sequences,

a, b, c

$$\frac{1}{b+c},\frac{1}{a+c},\frac{1}{a+b}$$

by the rearrangement inequality, we have

$$\begin{array}{ccc} a & b & c \\ \downarrow & \downarrow & \downarrow \\ \frac{1}{b+c} & \frac{1}{c+a} & \frac{1}{a+b} \end{array} \qquad \begin{array}{cccc} a & b & c & a \\ \searrow & \searrow & \searrow & \\ \frac{1}{b+c} & \frac{1}{c+a} & \frac{1}{a+b} & \frac{1}{b+c} \end{array}$$

$$\frac{a}{b+c}+\frac{b}{a+c}+\frac{c}{a+b}\geq\frac{a}{a+c}+\frac{b}{a+b}+\frac{c}{b+c} \qquad (1)$$

$$\begin{array}{ccc} a & b & c \\ \downarrow & \downarrow & \downarrow \\ \frac{1}{b+c} & \frac{1}{c+a} & \frac{1}{a+b} \end{array} \qquad \begin{array}{cccc} a & b & c & a \\ \nearrow & \nearrow & \nearrow & \\ \frac{1}{b+c} & \frac{1}{c+a} & \frac{1}{a+b} & \frac{1}{b+c} \end{array}$$

$$\frac{a}{b+c}+\frac{b}{a+c}+\frac{c}{a+b}\geq\frac{b}{b+c}+\frac{c}{a+c}+\frac{a}{a+b} \qquad (2)$$

$$(1)+(2):\ 2\left(\frac{a}{b+c}+\frac{b}{a+c}+\frac{c}{a+b}\right)\geq\frac{a+c}{a+c}+\frac{b+a}{a+b}+\frac{c+b}{b+c}=3$$

That, is $\frac{a}{b+c}+\frac{b}{c+a}+\frac{c}{a+b}\geq\frac{3}{2}$

Example 7. For all positive numbers a, b and c, prove the inequality

$$\frac{a^2}{b+c}+\frac{b^2}{c+a}+\frac{c^2}{a+b}\geq\frac{a+b+c}{2}.$$

Solution:

Because of the symmetry, we may assume that $a \le b \le c$, $a^2 \le b^2 \le c^2$, and $\frac{1}{b+c} \le \frac{1}{a+c} \le \frac{1}{a+b}$.

For the following two similarly ordered sequences,

$a^2, \quad b^2, \quad c^2$

$\frac{1}{b+c}, \quad \frac{1}{a+c}, \quad \frac{1}{a+b}$

by the rearrangement inequality,

$$\begin{matrix} a^2 & b^2 & c^2 \\ \downarrow & \downarrow & \downarrow \\ \frac{1}{b+c} & \frac{1}{c+a} & \frac{1}{a+b} \end{matrix} \qquad \begin{matrix} a^2 & & b^2 & & c^2 & & a^2 \\ & \searrow & & \searrow & & \searrow & \\ \frac{1}{b+c} & & \frac{1}{c+a} & & \frac{1}{a+b} & & \frac{1}{b+c} \end{matrix}$$

or

$$\begin{bmatrix} a^2 & b^2 & c^2 \\ \frac{1}{b+c} & \frac{1}{c+a} & \frac{1}{a+b} \end{bmatrix} \ge \begin{bmatrix} a^2 & b^2 & c^2 \\ \frac{1}{c+a} & \frac{1}{a+b} & \frac{1}{b+c} \end{bmatrix}$$

$$\frac{a^2}{b+c} + \frac{b^2}{a+c} + \frac{c^2}{a+b} \ge \frac{a^2}{a+c} + \frac{b^2}{a+b} + \frac{c^2}{b+c} \qquad (1)$$

$$\begin{matrix} a^2 & b^2 & c^2 \\ \downarrow & \downarrow & \downarrow \\ \frac{1}{b+c} & \frac{1}{c+a} & \frac{1}{a+b} \end{matrix} \qquad \begin{matrix} a^2 & & b^2 & & c^2 & & a^2 \\ & \nearrow & & \nearrow & & \nearrow & \\ \frac{1}{b+c} & & \frac{1}{c+a} & & \frac{1}{a+b} & & \frac{1}{b+c} \end{matrix}$$

Or

$$\begin{bmatrix} a^2 & b^2 & c^2 \\ \frac{1}{b+c} & \frac{1}{c+a} & \frac{1}{a+b} \end{bmatrix} \ge \begin{bmatrix} a^2 & b^2 & c^2 \\ \frac{1}{a+b} & \frac{1}{b+c} & \frac{1}{c+a} \end{bmatrix}$$

$$\frac{a^2}{b+c} + \frac{b^2}{a+c} + \frac{c^2}{a+b} \ge \frac{a^2}{a+b} + \frac{b^2}{b+c} + \frac{c^2}{c+a} \qquad (2)$$

(1) + (2): $2(\frac{a^2}{b+c}+\frac{b^2}{a+c}+\frac{c^2}{a+b}) \ge \frac{a^2+c^2}{a+c}+\frac{b^2+a^2}{a+b}+\frac{c^2+b^2}{b+c}$

Using the inequality $\frac{x^2+y^2}{x+y} \ge \frac{x+y}{2}$ for real x, y, we have

$$\frac{a^2+c^2}{a+c}+\frac{b^2+a^2}{a+b}+\frac{c^2+b^2}{b+c} \ge \frac{a+c}{2}+\frac{b+a}{2}+\frac{c+a}{2} = a+b+c$$

$$\frac{a^2}{b+c}+\frac{b^2}{a+c}+\frac{c^2}{a+b} \ge \frac{a+b+c}{2}.$$

Example 8. Let a, b, $c > 0$ be real numbers. Prove the inequality

$$\frac{a^2+bc}{b+c}+\frac{b^2+ca}{c+a}+\frac{c^2+ab}{a+b} \ge a+b+c.$$

Solution:

Since the expression is a symmetric function of a, b and c, we can assume, without loss of generality, that $a \le b \le c$, $a^2 \le b^2 \le c^2$, and $\frac{1}{b+c} \le \frac{1}{a+c} \le \frac{1}{a+b}$.

Then we have the following two similarly ordered sequences:

$a^2 \le b^2 \le c^2$

$\frac{1}{b+c}, \frac{1}{a+c}, \frac{1}{a+b}$.

By the rearrangement inequality,

$$\begin{array}{ccc} a^2 & b^2 & c^2 \\ \downarrow & \downarrow & \downarrow \\ \frac{1}{b+c} & \frac{1}{a+c} & \frac{1}{a+b} \end{array} \qquad \begin{array}{cccc} a^2 & b^2 & c^2 & a^2 \\ \nearrow & \nearrow & \nearrow & \\ \frac{1}{b+c} & \frac{1}{a+c} & \frac{1}{a+b} & \frac{1}{b+c} \end{array}$$

$$\frac{a^2}{b+c}+\frac{b^2}{a+c}+\frac{c^2}{a+b} \ge \frac{b^2}{b+c}+\frac{c^2}{a+c}+\frac{a^2}{a+b} \qquad (1)$$

Add $\frac{bc}{b+c}+\frac{ca}{c+a}+\frac{ab}{a+b}$ to both sides of (1):

$$\frac{a^2}{b+c}+\frac{b^2}{a+c}+\frac{c^2}{a+b}+\frac{bc}{b+c}+\frac{ca}{c+a}+\frac{ab}{a+b}$$

$\geq \frac{b^2}{b+c} + \frac{c^2}{a+c} + \frac{a^2}{a+b} + \frac{bc}{b+c} + \frac{ca}{c+a} + \frac{ab}{a+b}$

$= (\frac{b^2}{b+c} + \frac{bc}{b+c}) + (\frac{c^2}{a+c} + \frac{ca}{c+a}) + (\frac{a^2}{a+b} + \frac{ab}{a+b})$

$= \frac{b^2+bc}{b+c} + \frac{c^2+ca}{a+c} + \frac{a^2+ab}{a+b} = \frac{b(b+c)}{b+c} + \frac{c(c+a)}{a+c} + \frac{a(c+b)}{a+b} = a + b + c.$

Example 9. Given that *a, b, c* are positive real numbers, prove $a + b + c \leq \frac{a^2+b^2}{2c} + \frac{b^2+c^2}{2a} + \frac{c^2+a^2}{2b} \leq \frac{a^3}{bc} + \frac{b^3}{ca} + \frac{c^3}{ab}$

Solution:

We prove this part first: $a + b + c \leq \frac{a^2+b^2}{2c} + \frac{b^2+c^2}{2a} + \frac{c^2+a^2}{2b}$.

Since the inequality is symmetric, WLOG, we may assume that $a \leq b \leq c$. Then we know that $a^2 \leq b^2 \leq c^2$.

Then we have the following two similarly ordered sequences:
a^2, b^2, c^2.
$\frac{1}{c} \leq \frac{1}{b} \leq \frac{1}{a}$

By the rearrangement inequality, we have

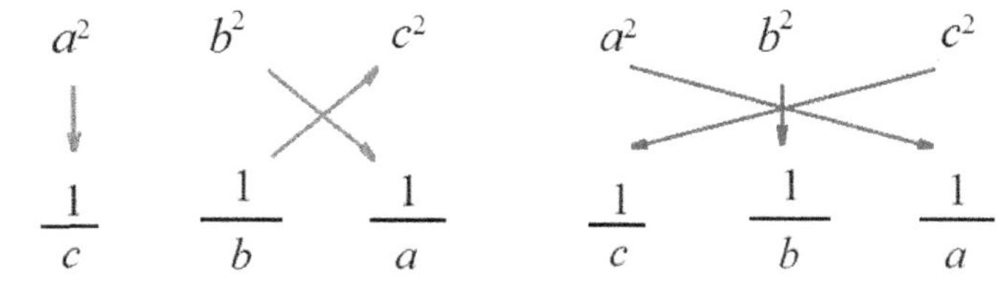

$a^2 \quad b^2 \quad c^2 \qquad\qquad a^2 \quad b^2 \quad c^2$

$\frac{1}{c} \quad \frac{1}{b} \quad \frac{1}{a} \qquad\qquad \frac{1}{c} \quad \frac{1}{b} \quad \frac{1}{a}$

$\frac{a^2}{c} + \frac{b^2}{a} + \frac{c^2}{b} \geq \frac{a^2}{a} + \frac{b^2}{b} + \frac{c^2}{c} = a + b + c$ (1)

$a^2 \quad b^2 \quad c^2 \qquad a^2 \quad b^2 \quad c^2$

$\frac{1}{c} \quad \frac{1}{b} \quad \frac{1}{a} \qquad \frac{1}{c} \quad \frac{1}{b} \quad \frac{1}{a}$

$$\frac{a^2}{b}+\frac{b^2}{c}+\frac{c^2}{a}\geq\frac{a^2}{a}+\frac{b^2}{b}+\frac{c^2}{c}=a+b+c \qquad (2)$$

(1) + (2):

$$\frac{a^2}{c}+\frac{b^2}{a}+\frac{c^2}{b}+\frac{a^2}{b}+\frac{b^2}{c}+\frac{c^2}{a}\geq 2(a+b+c)$$

$$\Rightarrow \qquad a+b+c\leq\frac{a^2+b^2}{2c}+\frac{b^2+c^2}{2a}+\frac{c^2+a^2}{2b}.$$

We prove $\frac{a^2+b^2}{2c}+\frac{b^2+c^2}{2a}+\frac{c^2+a^2}{2b}\leq\frac{a^3}{bc}+\frac{b^3}{ca}+\frac{c^3}{ab}$ then.

Then we have the following two similarly ordered sequences:

a^3, b^3, c^3.

$\frac{1}{bc}\leq\frac{1}{ac}\leq\frac{1}{ab}$

By the rearrangement inequality, we have

$a^3 \quad b^3 \quad c^3 \qquad a^3 \quad b^3 \quad c^3 \quad a^3$

$\frac{1}{bc} \quad \frac{1}{ac} \quad \frac{1}{ab} \qquad \frac{1}{bc} \quad \frac{1}{ac} \quad \frac{1}{ab} \quad \frac{1}{bc}$

$$\frac{a^3}{bc}+\frac{b^3}{ca}+\frac{c^3}{ab}\geq\frac{a^3}{ac}+\frac{b^3}{ab}+\frac{c^3}{bc} \qquad (3)$$

$a^3 \quad b^3 \quad c^3 \qquad a^3 \quad b^3 \quad c^3 \quad a^3$

$\frac{1}{bc} \quad \frac{1}{ac} \quad \frac{1}{ab} \qquad \frac{1}{bc} \quad \frac{1}{ac} \quad \frac{1}{ab} \quad \frac{1}{bc}$

$$\frac{a^3}{bc}+\frac{b^3}{ca}+\frac{c^3}{ab}\geq\frac{b^3}{bc}+\frac{c^3}{ca}+\frac{a^3}{ab} \qquad (4)$$

(3) + (4):

$$2\left(\frac{a^3}{bc}+\frac{b^3}{ca}+\frac{c^3}{ab}\right)\geq \frac{a^3}{ac}+\frac{b^3}{ab}+\frac{c^3}{bc}+\frac{b^3}{bc}+\frac{c^3}{ca}+\frac{a^3}{ab}$$

$$=\frac{a^2+b^2}{c}+\frac{b^2+c^2}{a}+\frac{c^2+a^2}{b} \qquad (5)$$

(5) ÷ 2: $\frac{a^2+b^2}{2c}+\frac{b^2+c^2}{2a}+\frac{c^2+a^2}{2b}\leq\frac{a^3}{bc}+\frac{b^3}{ca}+\frac{c^3}{ab}$.

Example 10. Prove that for all positive real numbers *a, b*, and *c*, $\frac{a^n}{bc}+\frac{b^n}{ca}+\frac{c^n}{ab}\geq a^{n-2}+b^{n-2}+c^{n-2}$.

Proof:

Since the inequality is symmetric, WLOG, we may assume that $a\leq b\leq c$. Then we know that $a^n\leq b^n\leq c^n$.

Then we have the following two similarly ordered sequences:

a^n, b^n, c^n

$\frac{1}{bc}, \frac{1}{ac}, \frac{1}{ab}$

By the rearrangement inequality, we have

$$\begin{matrix} a^n & b^n & c^n \\ \downarrow & \downarrow & \downarrow \\ \frac{1}{bc} & \frac{1}{ac} & \frac{1}{ab} \end{matrix} \qquad \begin{matrix} a^n & & b^n & & c^n & & a^n \\ & \searrow & & \searrow & & \searrow & \\ \frac{1}{bc} & & \frac{1}{ac} & & \frac{1}{ab} & & \frac{1}{bc} \end{matrix}$$

$$\frac{a^n}{bc}+\frac{b^n}{ca}+\frac{c^n}{ab}\geq\frac{a^n}{ac}+\frac{b^n}{ab}+\frac{c^n}{bc}=\frac{a^{n-1}}{c}+\frac{b^{n-1}}{a}+\frac{c^{n-1}}{b} \qquad (1)$$

Then we have the following two similarly ordered sequences:

$a^{n-1}, b^{n-1}, c^{n-1}$

$\frac{1}{c}, \frac{1}{b}, \frac{1}{a}$

By the rearrangement inequality, we have

a^{n-1} b^{n-1} c^{n-1} $\quad$ a^{n-1} b^{n-1} c^{n-1}

$\frac{1}{c}$ $\frac{1}{b}$ $\frac{1}{a}$ $\quad$ $\frac{1}{c}$ $\frac{1}{b}$ $\frac{1}{a}$

$$\frac{a^{n-1}}{c}+\frac{b^{n-1}}{a}+\frac{c^{n-1}}{b}\geq \frac{a^{n-1}}{a}+\frac{c^{n-1}}{c}+\frac{b^{n-1}}{b}=a^{n-2}+b^{n-2}+c^{n-2}\ .$$

$$\frac{a^4}{c}+\frac{b^4}{a}+\frac{c^4}{b}\geq \frac{a^4}{a}+\frac{c^4}{c}+\frac{b^4}{b}=a^3+b^3+c^3\ .$$

Example 11. a, b and c are three positive real numbers with $abc = 1$. Prove $a^3 + b^3 + c^3 + (ab)^3 + (bc)^3 + (ca)^3 \geq 2(a^2b + b^2c + c^2a)$.

Solution:

Since the expression $a^3 + b^3 + c^3 + (ab)^3 + (bc)^3 + (ca)^3$ is a symmetric function of a, b, and c, we can assume, without loss of generality, that $a \leq b \leq c$, $a^2 \leq b^2 \leq c^2$, $\frac{1}{c}\leq\frac{1}{b}\leq\frac{1}{a}$, and $\frac{1}{c^2}\leq\frac{1}{b^2}\leq\frac{1}{a^2}$

Then we have the following two similarly ordered sequences:

$a,\ b,\ c$

$a^2,\ b^2,\ c^2$.

By the rearrangement inequality, we have

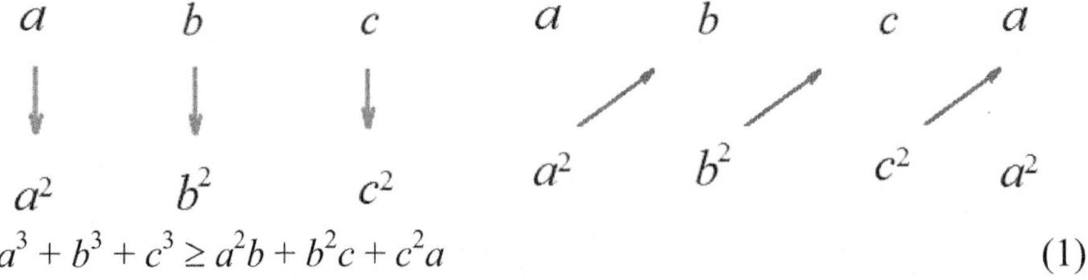

$$a^3 + b^3 + c^3 \geq a^2b + b^2c + c^2a \qquad (1)$$

Then we have the following two similarly ordered sequences:

$\frac{1}{c},\frac{1}{b},\frac{1}{a}$

$\frac{1}{c^2},\frac{1}{b^2},\frac{1}{a^2}$

By the rearrangement inequality, we have

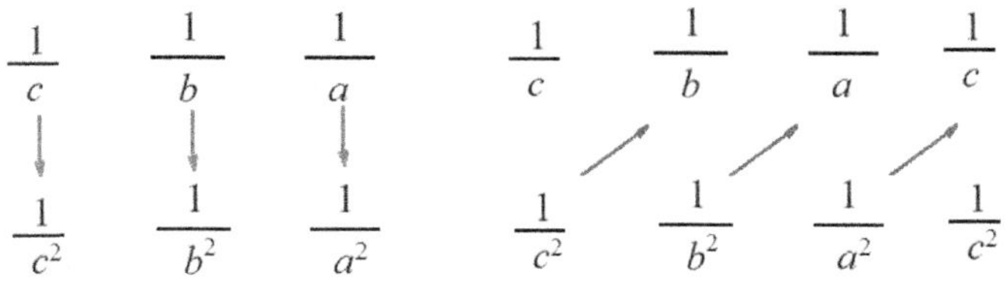

$$\begin{matrix} \frac{1}{c} & \frac{1}{b} & \frac{1}{a} \\ \downarrow & \downarrow & \downarrow \\ \frac{1}{c^2} & \frac{1}{b^2} & \frac{1}{a^2} \end{matrix} \qquad \begin{matrix} \frac{1}{c} & & \frac{1}{b} & & \frac{1}{a} & & \frac{1}{c} \\ & \nearrow & & \nearrow & & \nearrow & \\ \frac{1}{c^2} & & \frac{1}{b^2} & & \frac{1}{a^2} & & \frac{1}{c^2} \end{matrix}$$

$$(ab)^3 + (bc)^3 + (ca)^3 = \frac{1}{c^3} + \frac{1}{b^3} + \frac{1}{a^3}$$

$$\geq \frac{1}{c^2} \cdot \frac{1}{b} + \frac{1}{b^2} \cdot \frac{1}{a} + \frac{1}{a^2} \cdot \frac{1}{c} = \frac{a}{c} + \frac{c}{b} + \frac{b}{a} = a^2b + b^2c + c^2a \qquad (2)$$

(1) + (2): $a^3 + b^3 + c^3 + (ab)^3 + (bc)^3 + (ca)^3 \geq 2(a^2b + b^2c + c^2a)$.

Example 12. If a, b and c are positive real numbers, show that
$$\frac{a^4}{b^3+c^3} + \frac{b^4}{c^3+a^3} + \frac{c^4}{a^3+b^3} \geq \frac{a+b+c}{2}.$$

Solution:
So the expression is a symmetric function of a, b, and c. Then we can assume, without loss of generality, that $a \leq b \leq c \leq$. Thus, we know that
$a^4 \leq b^4 \leq c^4$ and $\frac{1}{b^3+c^3} \leq \frac{1}{c^3+a^3} \leq \frac{1}{a^3+b^3}$.

Then we have the following two similarly ordered sequences:
a^4, b^4, c^4
$$\frac{1}{b^3 + c^3}, \frac{1}{c^3 + a^3}, \frac{1}{a^3 + b^3}$$

By the rearrangement inequality,

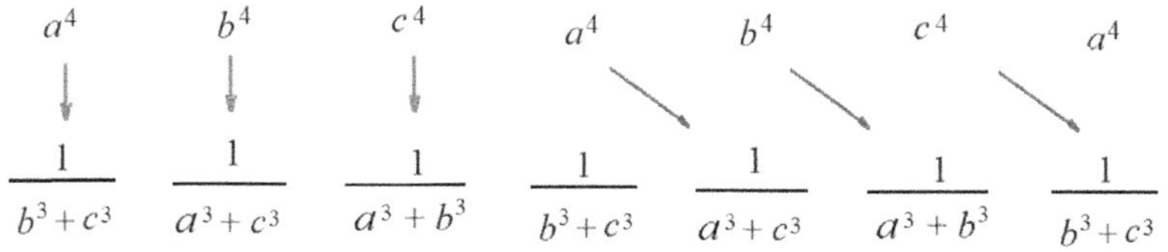

$$\begin{matrix} a^4 & b^4 & c^4 \\ \downarrow & \downarrow & \downarrow \\ \frac{1}{b^3+c^3} & \frac{1}{a^3+c^3} & \frac{1}{a^3+b^3} \end{matrix} \qquad \begin{matrix} a^4 & & b^4 & & c^4 & & a^4 \\ & \searrow & & \searrow & & \searrow & \\ \frac{1}{b^3+c^3} & & \frac{1}{a^3+c^3} & & \frac{1}{a^3+b^3} & & \frac{1}{b^3+c^3} \end{matrix}$$

$$\frac{a^4}{b^3+c^3} + \frac{b^4}{c^3+a^3} + \frac{c^4}{a^3+b^3} \geq \frac{c^4}{b^3+c^3} + \frac{a^4}{c^3+a^3} + \frac{b^4}{a^3+b^3} \qquad (1)$$

$$\begin{array}{ccccccc} a^4 & b^4 & c^4 & a^4 & b^4 & c^4 & a^4 \\ \downarrow & \downarrow & \downarrow & \nearrow & \nearrow & \nearrow & \\ \frac{1}{b^3+c^3} & \frac{1}{a^3+c^3} & \frac{1}{a^3+b^3} & \frac{1}{b^3+c^3} & \frac{1}{a^3+c^3} & \frac{1}{a^3+b^3} & \frac{1}{b^3+c^3} \end{array}$$

$$\frac{a^4}{b^3+c^3}+\frac{b^4}{c^3+a^3}+\frac{c^4}{a^3+b^3} \geq \frac{b^4}{b^3+c^3}+\frac{c^4}{c^3+a^3}+\frac{a^4}{a^3+b^3} \qquad (2)$$

(1) + (2):

$$2\left(\frac{a^4}{b^3+c^3}+\frac{b^4}{c^3+a^3}+\frac{c^4}{a^3+b^3}\right) \geq \frac{b^4+c^4}{b^3+c^3}+\frac{c^4+a^4}{c^3+a^3}+\frac{a^4+b^4}{a^3+b^3} \qquad (3)$$

Now we will prove that: $\frac{a^4+b^4}{a^3+b^3} \geq \frac{a+b}{2}$ $\Leftrightarrow 2(a^4+b^4) \geq (a^3+b^3)(a+b)$
$\Leftrightarrow a^4+b^4 \geq a^3b+b^3a.$

For the following two similarly ordered sequences:
$a,\ b,\ c$
$a^3,\ b^3,\ c^3,$

By the rearrangement inequality,

$$\begin{array}{cc} a & b \\ \downarrow & \downarrow \\ a^3 & b^3 \end{array} \qquad \begin{array}{cc} a & b \\ \times & \\ a^3 & b^3 \end{array}$$

We have $a^4+b^4 \geq a^3b+b^3a$. Thus $\frac{a^4+b^4}{a^3+b^3} \geq \frac{a+b}{2}$.

Similarly $\frac{b^4+c^4}{b^3+c^3} \geq \frac{b+c}{2}$, and $\frac{c^4+a^4}{c^3+a^3} \geq \frac{c+a}{2}$.
Therefore,

$$2\left(\frac{a^4}{b^3+c^3}+\frac{b^4}{c^3+a^3}+\frac{c^4}{a^3+b^3}\right) \geq \frac{b+c}{2}+\frac{c+a}{2}+\frac{a+b}{2} = a+b+c$$

or $\frac{a^4}{b^3+c^3}+\frac{b^4}{c^3+a^3}+\frac{c^4}{a^3+b^3} \geq \frac{a+b+c}{2}$.

CHAPER 4. PROBLEMS

Problem 1. Is the expression $\frac{a^2}{b+c}+\frac{b^2}{c+a}+\frac{c^2}{a+b}$ symmetric?

Problem 2. Is the expression Symmetric? $\frac{a^2+c^2}{b}+\frac{b^2+a^2}{c}+\frac{c^2+a^2}{a}$.

Problem 3. Prove that for all positive real numbers *a, b, c,* $\frac{ab}{c}+\frac{bc}{a}+\frac{ca}{b}\geq a+b+c$.

Problem 4. If $a, b, c > 0$ and $abc = 1$, show that
$\frac{1}{a^2(b+c)}+\frac{1}{b^2(a+c)}+\frac{1}{c^2(a+b)}\geq\frac{3}{2}$.

Problem 5. For all positive numbers *a, b* and *c*, prove the inequality
$\frac{a^2}{b^2+c^2}+\frac{b^2}{c^2+a^2}+\frac{c^2}{a^2+b^2}\geq\frac{3}{2}$.

Problem 6. For all positive numbers *a, b* and *c*, prove the inequality
$\frac{a^3b}{c}+\frac{a^3c}{b}+\frac{b^3a}{c}+\frac{b^3c}{a}+\frac{c^3a}{b}+\frac{c^3b}{a}\geq 6abc.$

Problem 7. Given that *a, b, c* are positive real numbers, prove
$\frac{b^3c^3+c^3a^3+a^3b^3}{abc}\geq 3abc.$

Problem 8. Prove that for all positive real numbers *a, b*, and *c*, $\frac{a^5}{bc}+\frac{b^5}{ca}+\frac{c^5}{ab}\geq a^3+b^3+c^3$.

Problem 9. Show that for positive real numbers *a, b, c*, $(a^2b + b^2c + c^2a)(ab^2 + bc^2 + ca^2 \geq 9a^2b^2c^2$.

Problem 10. Let $a, b, c > 0$ be real numbers. Prove the inequality

$$\frac{a^2-c^2}{b+c}+\frac{b^2-a^2}{c+a}+\frac{c^2-b^2}{a+b}\geq 0.$$

Problem 11. If a, b and c are positive real numbers, show that

$$\frac{a^4}{b^2+c^2}+\frac{b^4}{c^2+a^2}+\frac{c^4}{a^2+b^2}\geq\frac{a^2+b^2+c^2}{2}.$$

Problem 12. If a, b and c are the lengths of the sides of a triangle, prove that

$$\frac{a}{b+c-a}+\frac{b}{c+a-b}+\frac{c}{a+b-c}\geq 3.$$

Problem 13. Let a, b, c be positive real numbers. Prove the inequality $\frac{a}{2a+b+c}+$ $\frac{b}{a+2b+c}+\frac{c}{a+b+2c}\leq\frac{3}{4}.$

CHAPER 4. SOLUTIONS

Problem 1. Solution: Yes.

If we change a for b, we have $\frac{b^2}{a+c}+\frac{a^2}{c+b}+\frac{c^2}{b+a}$ which is the same as the given expression. So this expression is symmetric.

Problem 2. Solution: No.

We do the following replacements:

$a \Leftrightarrow b$, and we get $\frac{b^2+c^2}{a}+\frac{a^2+b^2}{c}+\frac{c^2+b^2}{b}$

We see that the new expression is different from the given one. So it is not symmetric.

Problem 3. Solution:

Method 1:

Since the expression is symmetric, WLOG, we can assume that $a \le b \le c$, we know that $ab \le ac \le bc$,

$$\frac{1}{c} \le \frac{b}{b} \le \frac{1}{a}$$

Then we have the following two similarly ordered sequences:

$ab, ca, bc,$

$\frac{1}{c}, \frac{1}{b}, \frac{1}{a}.$

By the rearrangement inequality, we have

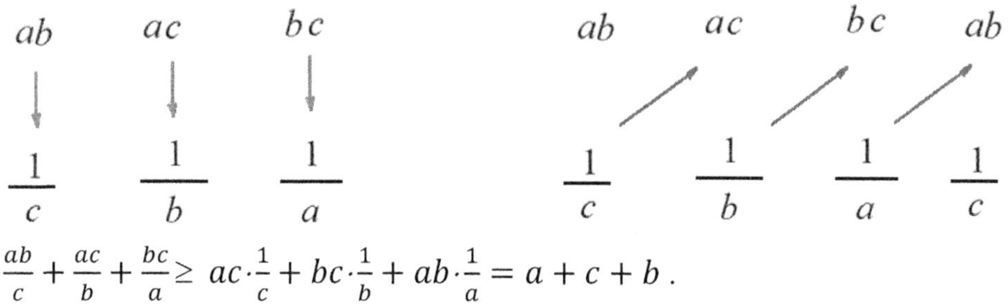

$$\frac{ab}{c}+\frac{ac}{b}+\frac{bc}{a} \ge ac \cdot \frac{1}{c} + bc \cdot \frac{1}{b} + ab \cdot \frac{1}{a} = a + c + b\ .$$

Method 2:

$$\frac{ab}{c}+\frac{bc}{a}+\frac{ca}{b}=\frac{1}{2}\left(\frac{ab}{c}+\frac{bc}{a}\right)+\frac{1}{2}\left(\frac{bc}{a}+\frac{ca}{b}\right)+\frac{1}{2}\left(\frac{ca}{b}+\frac{ab}{c}\right)$$

By AM-GM, $\frac{1}{2}\left(\frac{ab}{c}+\frac{bc}{a}\right)\geq\sqrt{\frac{ab}{c}\cdot\frac{bc}{a}}=b.$

$\frac{1}{2}\left(\frac{bc}{a}+\frac{ca}{b}\right)\geq\sqrt{\frac{bc}{a}\cdot\frac{ca}{b}}=c$, and $\frac{1}{2}\left(\frac{ca}{b}+\frac{ab}{c}\right)\geq\sqrt{\frac{ca}{b}\cdot\frac{ab}{c}}=a$

Adding these three inequalities we get:

$$\frac{ab}{c}+\frac{ac}{b}+\frac{bc}{a}\geq a+c+b\,.$$

Problem 4. Solution:

Let $x=\frac{1}{a}$, $y=\frac{1}{b}$, $z=\frac{1}{c}$. Then we have $xyz=1$. $x+y+z\geq 3$.

The original inequality can be written as

$$\frac{x}{y+z}+\frac{y}{z+x}+\frac{z}{x+y}\geq\frac{3}{2}.$$

By the symmetrical property, we assume that $x\leq y\leq z$

Then we have $x\leq y\leq z$ and $\frac{1}{y+z}\leq\frac{1}{z+x}\leq\frac{1}{x+y}$

For the following similarly ordered sequences,

$x,\ y,\ z$

$\frac{1}{y+z},\frac{1}{z+x},\frac{1}{x+y}$

based on the rearrangement inequality,

$$\begin{array}{ccccccc} x & y & z & x & y & z & x \\ \downarrow & \downarrow & \downarrow & \searrow & \searrow & \searrow & \\ \frac{1}{y+z} & \frac{1}{x+z} & \frac{1}{x+y} & \frac{1}{y+z} & \frac{1}{x+z} & \frac{1}{x+y} & \frac{1}{y+z} \end{array}$$

$$\frac{x}{y+z}+\frac{y}{z+x}+\frac{z}{x+y} \geq \frac{z}{y+z}+\frac{x}{z+x}+\frac{y}{x+y} \qquad (1)$$

$$\begin{array}{ccccccc} x & y & z & x & y & z & x \\ \downarrow & \downarrow & \downarrow & \nearrow & \nearrow & \nearrow & \\ \frac{1}{y+z} & \frac{1}{x+z} & \frac{1}{x+y} & \frac{1}{y+z} & \frac{1}{x+z} & \frac{1}{x+y} & \frac{1}{y+z} \end{array}$$

$$\frac{x}{y+z}+\frac{y}{z+x}+\frac{z}{x+y} \geq \frac{y}{y+z}+\frac{z}{z+x}+\frac{x}{x+y} \qquad (2)$$

(1) + (2): $2\left(\frac{x}{y+z}+\frac{y}{z+x}+\frac{z}{x+y}\right) \geq \frac{y+z}{y+z}+\frac{z+x}{z+x}+\frac{x+y}{x+y}=3$ (3)

(3) ÷ 2:

We get $\frac{x}{y+z}+\frac{y}{z+x}+\frac{z}{x+y} \geq \frac{3}{2}$. QED.

Problem 5. Solution:

Because of the symmetry, we may assume that $a \leq b \leq c$, $a^2 \leq b^2 \leq c^2$, and $\frac{1}{b^2+c^2} \leq \frac{1}{a^2+c^2} \leq \frac{1}{a^2+b^2}$.

For the following two similarly ordered sequences,

a^2, b^2, c^2

$\frac{1}{b^2+c^2}$, $\frac{1}{a^2+c^2}$, $\leq \frac{1}{a^2+b^2}$.

by the rearrangement inequality, we have

$$\frac{a^2}{b^2+c^2}+\frac{b^2}{c^2+a^2}+\frac{c^2}{a^2+b^2} \geq \frac{c^2}{b^2+c^2}+\frac{a^2}{c^2+a^2}+\frac{b^2}{a^2+b^2} \qquad (1)$$

$$\begin{array}{ccccccc} a^2 & b^2 & c^2 & a^2 & b^2 & c^2 & a^2 \\ \downarrow & \downarrow & \downarrow & \searrow & \searrow & \searrow & \\ \frac{1}{b^2+c^2} & \frac{1}{a^2+c^2} & \frac{1}{a^2+b^2} & \frac{1}{b^2+c^2} & \frac{1}{a^2+c^2} & \frac{1}{a^2+b^2} & \frac{1}{b^2+c^2} \end{array}$$

$$\frac{a^2}{b^2+c^2}+\frac{b^2}{c^2+a^2}+\frac{c^2}{a^2+b^2}\ge\frac{b^2}{b^2+c^2}+\frac{c^2}{c^2+a^2}+\frac{a^2}{a^2+b^2} \qquad (2)$$

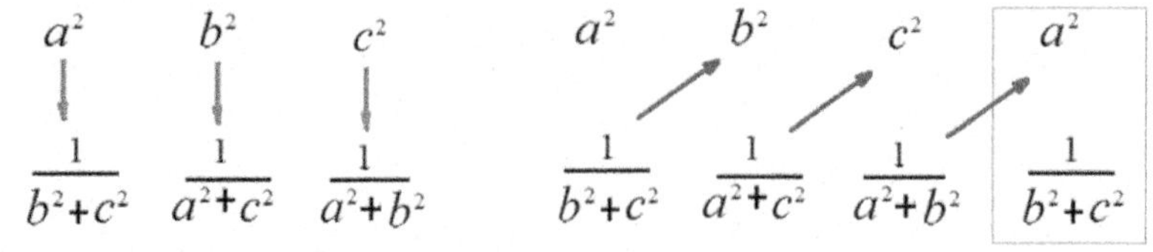

$a^2 \downarrow \frac{1}{b^2+c^2}$, $b^2 \downarrow \frac{1}{a^2+c^2}$, $c^2 \downarrow \frac{1}{a^2+b^2}$

a^2, b^2, c^2, a^2 ↗ $\frac{1}{b^2+c^2}$, $\frac{1}{a^2+c^2}$, $\frac{1}{a^2+b^2}$, $\frac{1}{b^2+c^2}$

(1) + (2): $2(\frac{a^2}{b^2+c^2}+\frac{b^2}{c^2+a^2}+\frac{c^2}{a^2+b^2})\ge\frac{b^2+c^2}{b^2+c^2}+\frac{c^2+a^2}{c^2+a^2}+\frac{a^2+b^2}{a^2+b^2}=3.$

That is $\frac{a^2}{b^2+c^2}+\frac{b^2}{c^2+a^2}+\frac{c^2}{a^2+b^2}\ge\frac{3}{2}$.

Problem 6. Solution:

Because of the symmetry of the expression $\frac{a^3b}{c}+\frac{a^3c}{b}+\frac{b^3a}{c}+\frac{b^3c}{a}+\frac{c^3a}{b}+\frac{c^3b}{a}$, we may assume that $a\le b\le c$.

To prove the given inequality is the same as to prove the following two inequalities.

$$\frac{b^3c}{a}+\frac{c^3a}{b}+\frac{a^3b}{c}\ge 3abc$$

$$\frac{c^3b}{a}+\frac{a^3c}{b}+\frac{b^3a}{c}\ge 3abc$$

For the following two similarly ordered sequences,

a^2b^2, a^2c^2, b^2c^2

$\frac{a}{bc}$, $\frac{b}{ac}$, $\frac{c}{ab}$

by the rearrangement inequality,

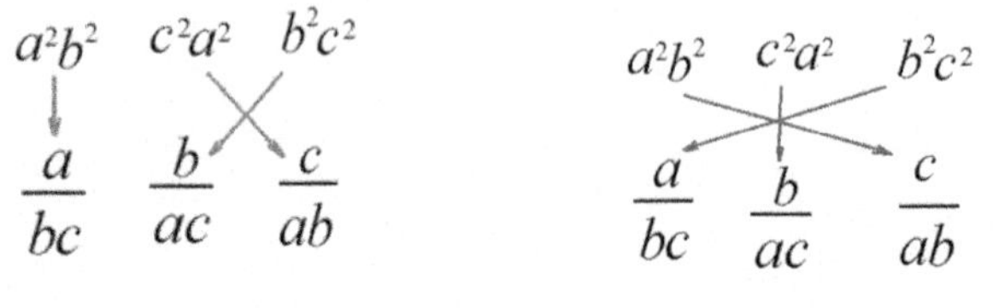

a^2b^2 c^2a^2 b^2c^2 → $\frac{a}{bc}$ $\frac{b}{ac}$ $\frac{c}{ab}$

a^2b^2 c^2a^2 b^2c^2 → $\frac{a}{bc}$ $\frac{b}{ac}$ $\frac{c}{ab}$

Or

$$\begin{bmatrix} a^2b^2 & b^2c^2 & c^2a^2 \\ \frac{a}{bc} & \frac{b}{ca} & \frac{c}{ab} \end{bmatrix} \ge \begin{bmatrix} a^2b^2 & b^2c^2 & c^2a^2 \\ \frac{c}{ab} & \frac{a}{bc} & \frac{b}{ca} \end{bmatrix}$$

$$\frac{a^2b^2a}{bc} + \frac{c^2a^2c}{ab} + \frac{b^2c^2b}{ac} = \frac{a^3b}{c} + \frac{c^3a}{b} + \frac{b^3c}{a}$$

$$\ge \frac{a^2b^2c}{ab} + \frac{b^2c^2a}{bc} + \frac{c^2a^2b}{ac} = 3abc \qquad (1)$$

$$\begin{array}{ccc} a^2b^2 & c^2a^2 & b^2c^2 \\ \frac{a}{bc} & \frac{b}{ac} & \frac{c}{ab} \end{array} \qquad \begin{array}{ccc} a^2b^2 & c^2a^2 & b^2c^2 \\ \frac{a}{bc} & \frac{b}{ac} & \frac{c}{ab} \end{array}$$

$$\begin{bmatrix} a^2b^2 & b^2c^2 & c^2a^2 \\ \frac{b}{ca} & \frac{c}{ab} & \frac{a}{bc} \end{bmatrix} \ge \begin{bmatrix} a^2b^2 & b^2c^2 & c^2a^2 \\ \frac{c}{ab} & \frac{a}{bc} & \frac{b}{ca} \end{bmatrix}$$

$$\frac{a^2b^2b}{ac} + \frac{c^2a^2c}{ab} + \frac{b^2c^2a}{bc} = \frac{b^3a}{c} + \frac{a^3c}{b} + \frac{c^3b}{a}$$
$$\ge \frac{a^2b^2c}{ab} + \frac{b^2c^2a}{bc} + \frac{c^2a^2b}{ac} = 3abc \qquad (2)$$

(1) + (2): $\frac{a^3b}{c} + \frac{a^3c}{b} + \frac{b^3a}{c} + \frac{b^3c}{a} + \frac{c^3a}{b} + \frac{c^3b}{a} \ge 6abc.$

Problem 7. Solution:

We write the given inequality as $\frac{b^3c^3+c^3a^3+a^3b^3}{abc} \ge 3abc.$

or

$$\frac{a^2b^2}{c} + \frac{c^2a^2}{b} + \frac{b^2c^2}{a} \ge 3abc$$

Since the inequality is symmetric, WLOG, we may assume that $a \le b \le c$.

Then we have the following two similarly ordered sequences,

$a^2b^2 \le c^2a^2 \le b^2c^2$

$\frac{1}{c} \le \frac{1}{b} \le \frac{1}{a}$

Then we have the following two similarly ordered sequences,

a^2b^2, c^2a^2, b^2c^2

$\frac{1}{c}, \frac{1}{b}, \frac{1}{a}$

$a^2b^2 \quad a^2c^2 \quad c^2b^2 \qquad a^2b^2 \quad a^2c^2 \quad c^2b^2 \quad a^2b^2$

$\frac{1}{c} \quad \frac{1}{b} \quad \frac{1}{a} \qquad \frac{1}{c} \quad \frac{1}{b} \quad \frac{1}{a} \quad \frac{1}{c}$

By the rearrangement inequality, we have

$$\frac{a^2b^2}{c} + \frac{c^2a^2}{b} + \frac{b^2c^2}{a} \ge a^2c + c^2b + ab^2$$

For the following two similarly ordered sequences:

$a, b, c,$

$ab, ca, bc,$

by the rearrangement inequality, we have

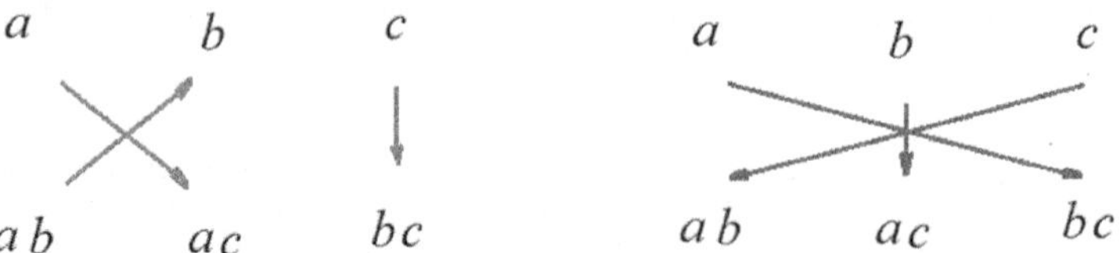

$$a^2c + c^2b + ab^2 \ge abc + bac + abc = 3abc.$$

Thus $\frac{b^3c^3+c^3a^3+a^3b^3}{abc} \ge \frac{a^2b^2}{c} + \frac{c^2a^2}{b} + \frac{b^2c^2}{a} \ge a^2c + c^2b + ab^2 \ge 3abc$

Problem 8. Proof:

Since the inequality is symmetric, WLOG, we may assume that $a \le b \le c$. Then we know that $a^5 \le b^5 \le c^5$.

Then we have the following two similarly ordered sequences:
a^5, b^5, c^5.
$\frac{1}{bc}, \frac{1}{ac}, \frac{1}{ab}$

By the rearrangement inequality, we have

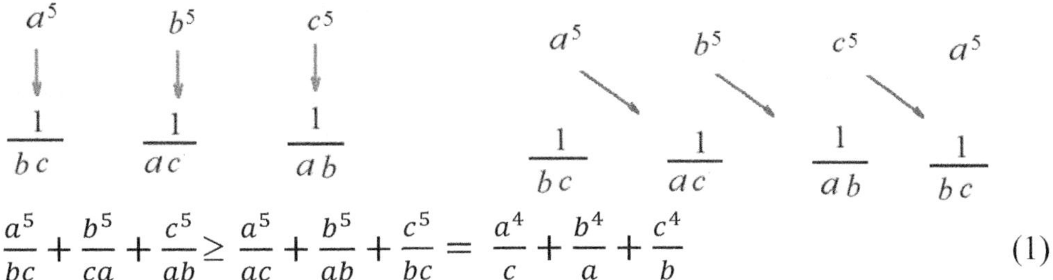

$$\frac{a^5}{bc} + \frac{b^5}{ca} + \frac{c^5}{ab} \geq \frac{a^5}{ac} + \frac{b^5}{ab} + \frac{c^5}{bc} = \frac{a^4}{c} + \frac{b^4}{a} + \frac{c^4}{b} \qquad (1)$$

Then we have the following two similarly ordered sequences:
a^4, b^4, c^4.
$\frac{1}{c}, \frac{1}{b}, \frac{1}{a}$

By the rearrangement inequality, we have

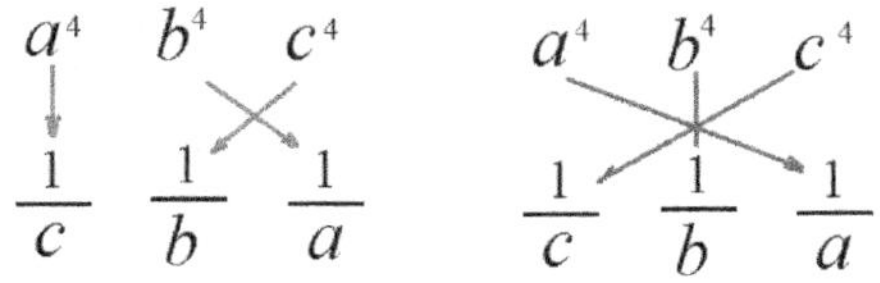

$$\frac{a^4}{c} + \frac{b^4}{a} + \frac{c^4}{b} \geq \frac{a^4}{a} + \frac{c^4}{c} + \frac{b^4}{b} = a^3 + b^3 + c^3$$

Problem 9. Solution:

Since the expression is a symmetric function of a, b and c, we can assume, without loss of generality, that $a \le b \le c$, $ab \le ac \le bc$, $a^2 \le b^2 \le c^2$.
Then we have the following two similarly ordered sequences:
a, b, c
ab, ac, bc.

By the rearrangement inequality,

$a \quad b \quad c \qquad a \quad b \quad c$

$ab \quad ac \quad bc \qquad ab \quad ac \quad bc$

$a^2b + b^2c + c^2a \ge abc + bac + cab = 3abc$ (1)

Then we have the following two similarly ordered sequences:

$a,\ b,\ c$

$a^2,\ b^2,\ c^2.$

By the rearrangement inequality,

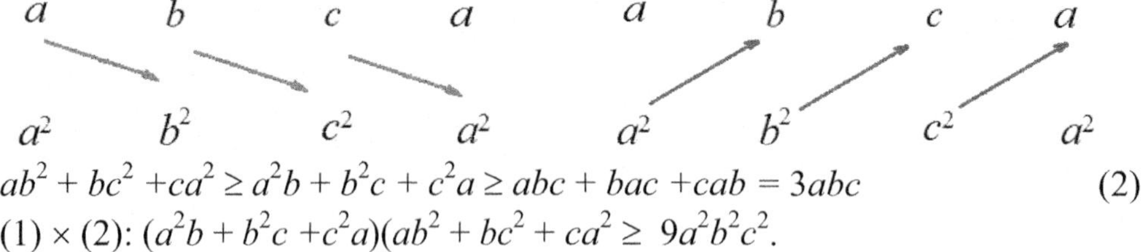

$ab^2 + bc^2 + ca^2 \ge a^2b + b^2c + c^2a \ge abc + bac + cab = 3abc$ (2)

(1) × (2): $(a^2b + b^2c + c^2a)(ab^2 + bc^2 + ca^2 \ge 9a^2b^2c^2.$

Problem 10. Solution:

The given inequality is equivalent to the following inequality:

$$\frac{a^2}{b+c} + \frac{b^2}{c+a} + \frac{c^2}{a+b} \ge \frac{c^2}{b+c} + \frac{a^2}{c+a} + \frac{b^2}{a+b}.$$

Since the expression $\frac{a^2}{b+c} + \frac{b^2}{c+a} + \frac{c^2}{a+b}$ is a symmetric function of a, b and c, we can assume, without loss of generality, that $a \le b \le c$, $a^2 \le b^2 \le c^2$, and $\frac{1}{b+c} \le \frac{1}{a+c} \le \frac{1}{a+b}$.

Then we have the following two similarly ordered sequences:

$a^2 \le b^2 \le c^2$

$\frac{1}{b+c}, \frac{1}{a+c}, \frac{1}{a+b}.$

By the rearrangement inequality,

$$\begin{array}{ccc} a^2 & b^2 & c^2 \\ \downarrow & \downarrow & \downarrow \\ \frac{1}{b+c} & \frac{1}{a+c} & \frac{1}{a+b} \end{array} \qquad \begin{array}{cccc} a^2 & b^2 & c^2 & a^2 \\ \searrow & \searrow & \searrow & \\ \frac{1}{b+c} & \frac{1}{a+c} & \frac{1}{a+b} & \frac{1}{b+c} \end{array}$$

$$\frac{a^2}{b+c}+\frac{b^2}{c+a}+\frac{c^2}{a+b}\geq\frac{c^2}{b+c}+\frac{a^2}{c+a}+\frac{b^2}{a+b}.$$

Equality occurs if and only if $a = b = c$.

Problem 11. Solution:

So the expression is a symmetric function of a, b, and c. Then we can assume, without loss of generality, that $a \leq b \leq c \leq$. Thus, we know that $a^4 \leq b^4 \leq c^4$ and $\frac{1}{b^2+c^2} \leq \frac{1}{c^2+a^2} \leq \frac{1}{a^2+b^2}$.

Then we have the following two similarly ordered sequences:

a^4, b^4, c^4

$\frac{1}{b^2+c^2}, \frac{1}{c^2+a^2}, \frac{1}{a^2+b^2}$

By the rearrangement inequality,

$$\begin{array}{ccc} a^4 & b^4 & c^4 \\ \downarrow & \downarrow & \downarrow \\ \frac{1}{b^2+c^2} & \frac{1}{c^2+a^2} & \frac{1}{a^2+b^2} \end{array} \qquad \begin{array}{cccc} a^4 & b^4 & c^4 & a^4 \\ \searrow & \searrow & \searrow & \\ \frac{1}{b^2+c^2} & \frac{1}{c^2+a^2} & \frac{1}{a^2+b^2} & \frac{1}{b^2+c^2} \end{array}$$

$$\frac{a^4}{b^2+c^2}+\frac{b^4}{c^2+a^2}+\frac{c^4}{a^2+b^2}\geq\frac{c^4}{b^2+c^2}+\frac{a^4}{c^2+a^2}+\frac{b^4}{a^2+b^2} \qquad (1)$$

$$\begin{array}{ccc} a^4 & b^4 & c^4 \\ \downarrow & \downarrow & \downarrow \\ \frac{1}{b^2+c^2} & \frac{1}{c^2+a^2} & \frac{1}{a^2+b^2} \end{array} \qquad \begin{array}{cccc} a^4 & b^4 & c^4 & a^4 \\ \nearrow & \nearrow & \nearrow & \\ \frac{1}{b^2+c^2} & \frac{1}{c^2+a^2} & \frac{1}{a^2+b^2} & \frac{1}{b^2+c^2} \end{array}$$

$$\frac{a^4}{b^2+c^2}+\frac{b^4}{c^2+a^2}+\frac{c^4}{a^2+b^2}\geq\frac{b^4}{b^2+c^2}+\frac{c^4}{c^2+a^2}+\frac{a^4}{a^2+b^2} \quad (2)$$

(1) + (2):

$$2\left(\frac{a^4}{b^2+c^2}+\frac{b^4}{c^2+a^2}+\frac{c^4}{a^2+b^2}\right)\geq\frac{b^4+c^4}{b^2+c^2}+\frac{c^4+a^4}{c^2+a^2}+\frac{a^4+b^4}{a^2+b^2}$$

$$\geq\frac{b^2+c^2}{2}+\frac{c^2+a^2}{2}+\frac{a^2+b^2}{2}=a^2+b^2+c^2$$

or $\frac{a^4}{b^2+c^2}+\frac{b^4}{c^2+a^2}+\frac{c^4}{a^2+b^2}\geq\frac{a^2+b^2+c^2}{2}$.

Problem 12. Solution:

We see that when we exchange the positions of a and b, we get the same expression $\frac{b}{a+c-b}+\frac{a}{c+b-a}+\frac{c}{a+b-c}$.

So the expression is a symmetric function of a, b, and c. Then we can assume, without loss of generality, that $a\leq b\leq c$, $\frac{1}{b+c-a}\leq\frac{1}{c+a-b}\leq\frac{1}{a+b-c}$.

Then we have the following two similarly ordered sequences:

a, b, c

$\frac{1}{b+c-a}, \frac{1}{c+a-b}, \frac{1}{a+b-c}$

By the rearrangement inequality, we have

$$\begin{array}{ccc} a & b & c \\ \downarrow & \downarrow & \downarrow \\ \frac{1}{b+c-a} & \frac{1}{c+a-b} & \frac{1}{a+b-c} \end{array} \qquad \begin{array}{cccc} a & b & c & a \\ \searrow & \searrow & \searrow & \\ \frac{1}{b+c-a} & \frac{1}{c+a-b} & \frac{1}{a+b-c} & \frac{1}{b+c-a} \end{array}$$

$$\frac{a}{b+c-a}+\frac{b}{c+a-b}+\frac{c}{a+b-c}\geq\frac{c}{b+c-a}+\frac{a}{c+a-b}+\frac{b}{a+b-c} \quad (1)$$

$$\begin{array}{ccc} a & b & c \\ \downarrow & \downarrow & \downarrow \\ \frac{1}{b+c-a} & \frac{1}{c+a-b} & \frac{1}{a+b-c} \end{array} \qquad \begin{array}{cccc} a & b & c & a \\ \nearrow & \nearrow & \nearrow & \\ \frac{1}{b+c-a} & \frac{1}{c+a-b} & \frac{1}{a+b-c} & \frac{1}{b+c-a} \end{array}$$

$$\frac{a}{b+c-a}+\frac{b}{c+a-b}+\frac{c}{a+b-c} \geq \frac{b}{b+c-a}+\frac{c}{c+a-b}+\frac{a}{a+b-c} \qquad (2)$$

(1) + (2):

$$2\left(\frac{a}{b+c-a}+\frac{b}{c+a-b}+\frac{c}{a+b-c}\right) \geq \frac{b+c}{b+c-a}+\frac{c+a}{c+a-b}+\frac{a+b}{a+b-c}$$

Or $2\left(\frac{a}{b+c-a}+\frac{b}{c+a-b}+\frac{c}{a+b-c}\right) \geq \frac{b+c-a+a}{b+c-a}+\frac{c+a-b+b}{c+a-b}+\frac{a+b-c+c}{a+b-c}$

$$\Rightarrow 2\left(\frac{a}{b+c-a}+\frac{b}{c+a-b}+\frac{c}{a+b-c}\right) \geq 3+\frac{a}{b+c-a}+\frac{b}{c+a-b}+\frac{c}{a+b-c}$$

$\Rightarrow \frac{a}{b+c-a}+\frac{b}{c+a-b}+\frac{c}{a+b-c} \geq 3$. QED.

Problem 13. Solution:

Since the inequality is symmetrical, WLOG, we can assume that $a \leq b \leq c$, we have the following two similarly ordered sequences:

$a,\ b,\ c$

$\frac{1}{a+b+2c}, \frac{1}{a+2b+c}, \frac{1}{2a+b+c}$.

By the rearrangement inequality, we have

$$\frac{a}{2a+b+c}+\frac{b}{a+2b+c}+\frac{c}{a+b+2c} \leq \frac{a}{2a+b+c}+\frac{b}{a+2b+c}+\frac{c}{a+b+2c} \qquad (1)$$

(1) × 2:

$$2\left(\frac{a}{2a+b+c}+\frac{b}{a+2b+c}+\frac{c}{a+b+2c}\right) \leq \frac{2a}{2a+b+c}+\frac{2b}{a+2b+c}+\frac{2c}{a+b+2c} \qquad (2)$$

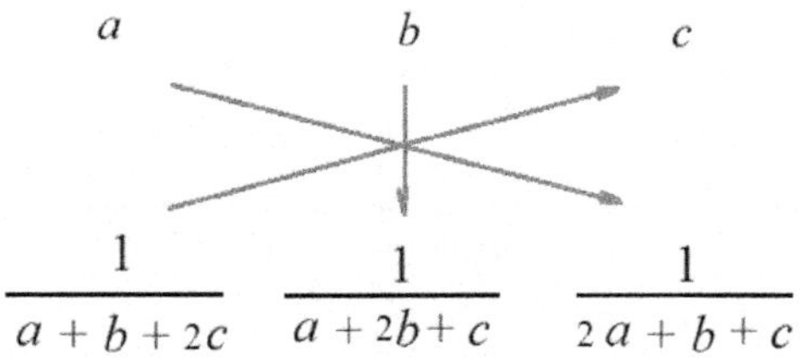

$a \quad b \quad c \qquad\qquad a \quad b \quad c$

$$\frac{1}{a+b+2c} \quad \frac{1}{a+2b+c} \quad \frac{1}{2a+b+c} \qquad\qquad \frac{1}{a+b+2c} \quad \frac{1}{a+2b+c} \quad \frac{1}{2a+b+c}$$

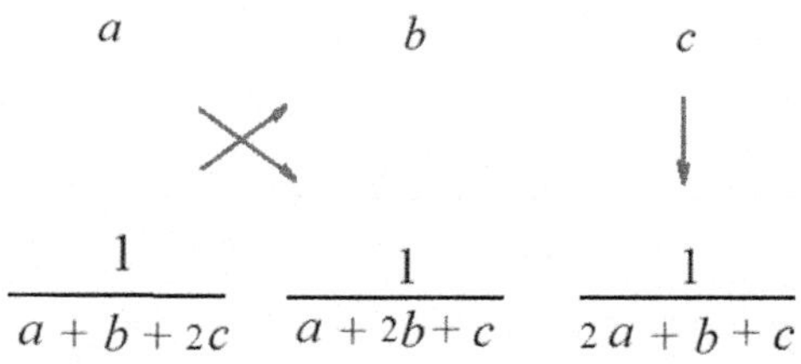

$$\frac{a}{2a+b+c}+\frac{b}{a+2b+c}+\frac{c}{a+b+2c} \le \frac{c}{2a+b+c}+\frac{a}{a+2b+c}+\frac{b}{a+b+2c} \qquad (3)$$

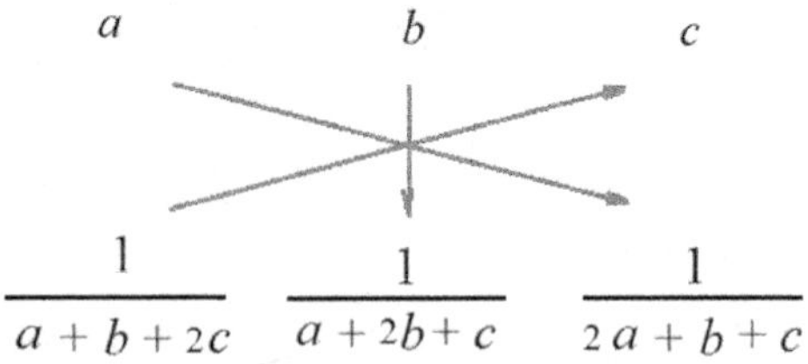

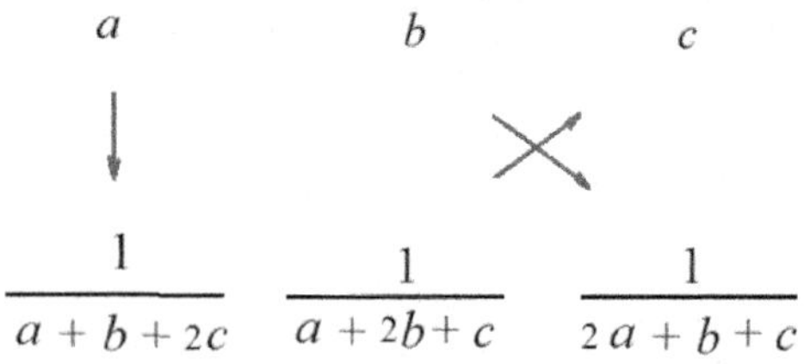

$a \quad b \quad c \qquad\qquad a \quad b \quad c$

$$\frac{1}{a+b+2c} \quad \frac{1}{a+2b+c} \quad \frac{1}{2a+b+c} \qquad\qquad \frac{1}{a+b+2c} \quad \frac{1}{a+2b+c} \quad \frac{1}{2a+b+c}$$

$$\frac{a}{2a+b+c}+\frac{b}{a+2b+c}+\frac{c}{a+b+2c} \le \frac{b}{2a+b+c}+\frac{c}{a+2b+c}+\frac{a}{a+b+2c} \qquad (4)$$

(2) + (3) + (4):

$$4\left(\frac{a}{2a+b+c}+\frac{b}{a+2b+c}+\frac{c}{a+b+2c}\right) \le \frac{2a+b+c}{2a+b+c}+\frac{2b+a+c}{a+2b+c}+\frac{2c+a+b}{a+b+2c} = 3.$$

Therefore $\frac{a}{2a+b+c}+\frac{b}{a+2b+c}+\frac{c}{a+b+2c} \le \frac{3}{4}$. QED.

Chapter 5. Solving Cyclic Inequalities

A cyclic polynomial is a polynomial that remains the same under cyclic permutation or rotation of the variables.

$f(a_1, a_2, \ldots a_n)$ is a cyclic expression in $a_1, a_2, \ldots a_n$ if, for $a_1 \Rightarrow a_2, a_2 \Rightarrow a_3, \ldots a_n \Rightarrow a_1$, we have $f(a_1, a_2, \ldots a_n) = f(a_n, a_{n-1}, \ldots, a_2, a_1)$.

Examples of cyclic expressions

$a^2 + b^2 + c^2$
$a^2b + b^2c + c^2a$
$ab^2 + bc^2 + ca^2$
$(a^2b + b^2c + c^2a)(ab^2 + bc^2 + ca^2 \geq 9a^2b^2c^2.$
$a^3b^2 + b^3a^2$
$a^3b + b^3c + c^3a$

$x^3 + y^3 + z^3 + 3xyz - x^4yz - xy^4z - xyz^4$
$\frac{a}{a+b} + \frac{b}{b+c} + \frac{c}{c+a}.$
$\frac{1}{a^3(b+c)} + \frac{1}{b^3(a+c)} + \frac{1}{c^3(a+b)}.$
$\frac{a^2}{b+c} + \frac{b^2}{c+a} + \frac{c^2}{a+b}.$

Cyclic, Non-Symmetric Inequalities

Since $f(x, y, z)$ is cyclic, WLOG, we may assume that $x = \min(x, y, z)$. Then we have two cases:
Case 1: $x \leq y \leq z$
Case 2: $x \leq z \leq y$.

We may also assume that $x = \max\{x, y, z\}$. There are two cases as well:
Case 1: $x \geq y \geq z$
Case 2: $x \geq z \geq y$.

A symmetric polynomial is cyclic but not vice versa. For example, $f(x, y, z) = x^2 y + y^2 z + z^2 x$ is cyclic but not symmetric.

The algebraic sum, difference, product and quotient of two cyclic (or symmetric) functions are cyclic (symmetric).

Example 1. Is the expression $\frac{a}{b}+\frac{b}{c}+\frac{c}{a}$ cyclic?

Solution: Yes.

If we change a for b, b for c, c for a, we have $\frac{b}{c}+\frac{c}{a}+\frac{a}{b}$ which is the same as the given expression. So this expression is cyclic (but not symmetric).

Example 2. Is the expression $\frac{a}{b+c}+\frac{b}{c+a}+\frac{c}{a+b}$ cyclic?

Solution: Yes.

If we change a for b, b for c, and c for a, we have $\frac{b}{c+a}+\frac{c}{a+b}+\frac{a}{b+c}$ which is the same as the given expression. So this expression is cyclic.

Example 3. Is the expression $\frac{a^3}{b+c+d}+\frac{b^3}{c+d+a}+\frac{c^3}{d+a+b}+\frac{d^3}{a+b+c}$ cyclic?

Solution: Yes.

If we change a for b, b for c, c for d and d for a, we have $\frac{b^3}{c+d+a}+\frac{c^3}{d+a+b}+\frac{d^3}{a+b+c}+\frac{a^3}{b+c+d}$ which is the same as the given expression. So this expression is cyclic.

Example 4. Is the expression $\frac{a^3}{bc}+\frac{b^3}{ca}+\frac{c^3}{ab}$ cyclic?

Solution: Yes.

If we change a for b, b for c, and c for a, we have $\frac{b^3}{ca} + \frac{c^3}{ab} + \frac{a^3}{bc}$ which is the same as the given expression. So this expression is cyclic.

Example 5. Is the expression $\frac{a^2}{b} + \frac{b^2}{c} + \frac{c^2}{a}$ cyclic?

Solution: Yes.

If we change a for b, b for c, and c for a, we have $\frac{a^2}{b} + \frac{b^2}{c} + \frac{c^2}{a}$ which is the same as the given expression. So this expression is cyclic.

Example 6. Is the expression $\frac{a^3b}{c} + \frac{a^3c}{b} + \frac{b^3a}{c} + \frac{b^3c}{a} + \frac{c^3a}{b} + \frac{c^3b}{a}$ cyclic?

Solution: Yes.

If we change a for b, b for c, and c for a, we have $\frac{a^3b}{c} + \frac{a^3c}{b} + \frac{b^3a}{c} + \frac{b^3c}{a} + \frac{c^3a}{b} + \frac{c^3b}{a}$ which is the same as the given expression. So this expression is cyclic.

Because of the symmetry of the expression $\frac{a^3b}{c} + \frac{a^3c}{b} + \frac{b^3a}{c} + \frac{b^3c}{a} + \frac{c^3a}{b} + \frac{c^3b}{a}$, we may assume that $a \le b \le c$.

Example 7. Prove that for all positive real numbers a, b, c, we have $\frac{a^3}{b^2} + \frac{b^3}{c^2} + \frac{c^3}{a^2} \ge a + b + c$.

Solution:

Method 1:

The expression is cyclic but not symmetric.

Let us assume that

Case 1: $a \le b \le c$.

Case 2: $a \le c \le b$.

For case 1, we can write the following two similarly ordered sequences:
a^3, b^3, c^3.
$\frac{1}{c^2}, \frac{1}{b^2}, \frac{1}{a^2}$

By the rearrangement inequality, we have

$\frac{a^3}{b^2} + \frac{b^3}{c^2} + \frac{c^3}{a^2} \ge a^3 \cdot \frac{1}{a^2} + b^3 \cdot \frac{1}{b^2} + c^3 \cdot \frac{1}{c^2} = a + b + c$. QED.
The case 2 can be dealt similarly.

Method 2:
From AM-GM, we have

$$\frac{a^3}{b^2} + 2b = \frac{a^3}{b^2} + b + b \ge 3\sqrt[3]{\frac{a^3}{b^2} \cdot b \cdot b} = 3a \qquad (1)$$

Similarly,

$$\frac{b^3}{c^2} + 2c \ge 3b \qquad (2)$$

$$\frac{c^3}{a^2} + 2a \ge 3a \qquad (3)$$

(1) + (2) + (3):

$$\frac{a^3}{b^2} + \frac{b^3}{c^2} + \frac{c^3}{a^2} + 2(a + b + c) \ge 3(a + b + c)$$

That is $\frac{a^3}{b^2} + \frac{b^3}{c^2} + \frac{c^3}{a^2} \ge a + b + c$.
Equality holds iff $a = b = c$.

Example 8. Let a, b, c be real numbers. Prove the inequality
$a^5 + b^5 + c^5 \geq a^4b + b^4c + c^4a.$

Solution:
Method 1:
Without loss of generality we may assume that $a \leq b \leq c$, and then clearly $a^4 \leq b^4 \leq c^4$ (since the given inequality is cyclic, we also need to consider the case when $a \leq c \leq b$, which is analogous).

Now by the rearrangement inequality we get the required inequality.

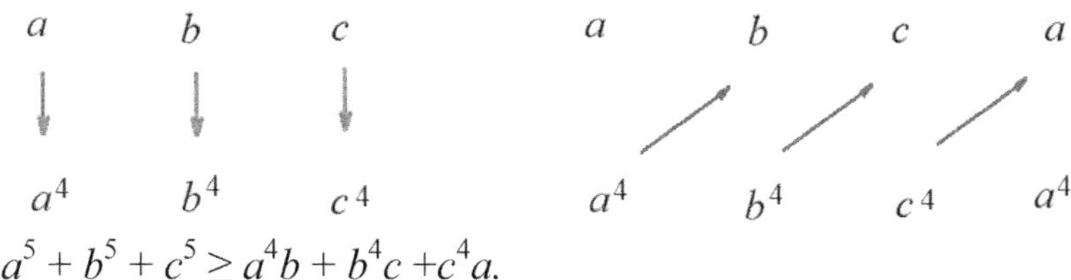

$a^5 + b^5 + c^5 \geq a^4b + b^4c + c^4a.$

Equality occurs iff $a = b = c$.

Method 2:
Since $AM \geq GM$ we obtain the following inequalities:
$a^5 + a^5 + a^5 + a^5 + b^5 \geq 5a4b,$
$b^5 + b^5 + b^5 + b^5 + c^5 \geq 5b4c,$
$c^5 + c^5 + c^5 + c^5 + a^5 \geq 5c4a,$
and adding the previous three inequalities yields required inequality. Equality occurs iff $a = b = c$.

Example 9. Let a, b, c be real numbers. Prove the inequality
$a^5 + b^5 + c^5 \geq a^3b^2 + b^3c^2 + c^3a^2.$

Solution:
Without loss of generality we may assume that $a \leq b \leq c$, and then clearly $a^2 \leq b^2 \leq c^2$, $a^3 \leq b^3 \leq c^3$ (since the given inequality is cyclic, we also need to consider the case when $a \leq c \leq b$, which is analogous).

Now by the rearrangement inequality we get the required inequality.

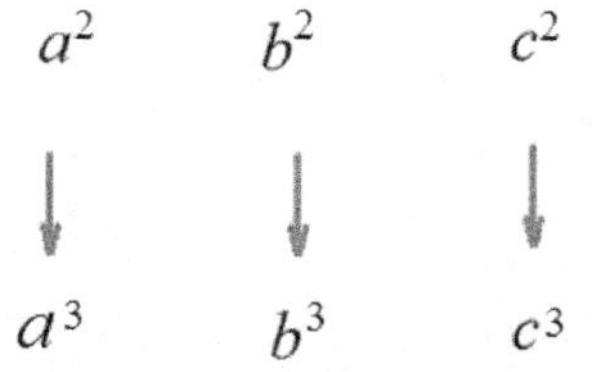

$a^2 \quad b^2 \quad c^2$

$\downarrow \quad \downarrow \quad \downarrow$

$a^3 \quad b^3 \quad c^3$

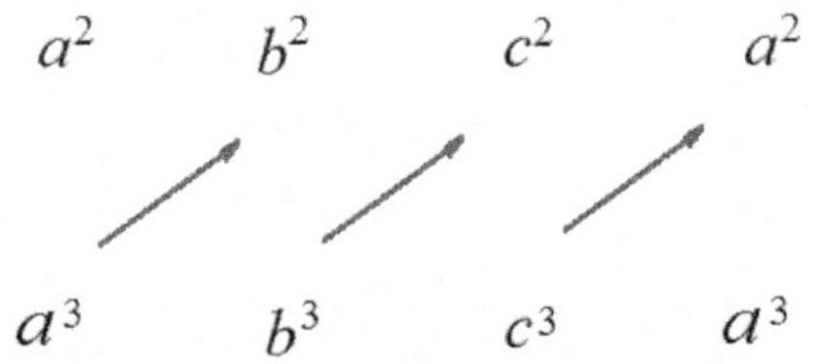

$a^2 \quad b^2 \quad c^2 \quad a^2$

$\nearrow \quad \nearrow \quad \nearrow$

$a^3 \quad b^3 \quad c^3 \quad a^3$

$a^5 + b^5 + c^5 \geq a^3b^2 + b^3c^2 + c^3a^2$.

Example 10. Show that $\frac{1}{b(a+b)} + \frac{1}{c(b+c)} + \frac{1}{a(c+a)} \geq \frac{1}{b(a+c)} + \frac{1}{c(b+a)} + \frac{1}{a(c+b)}$. a, b, c are positive real numbers.

Proof:
The given expression is not symmetric but cyclic. So we are not able to assume that $a \leq b \leq c$. However, we can, WLOG, assume that a is $\min\{a, b, c\}$.

Thus we have two cases: 1: $a \leq b \leq c$, and 2: $a \leq c \leq b$.

For case 1, $a \leq b \leq c$,
$\frac{1}{c} \leq \frac{1}{b} \leq \frac{1}{a}$. $\frac{1}{b+c} \leq \frac{1}{a+c} \leq \frac{1}{a+b}$.

For the two similarly sorted sequences
$\frac{1}{c}, \frac{1}{b}, \frac{1}{a}$
$\frac{1}{b+c}, \frac{1}{a+c}, \frac{1}{a+b}$
by the rearrangement inequality, we have

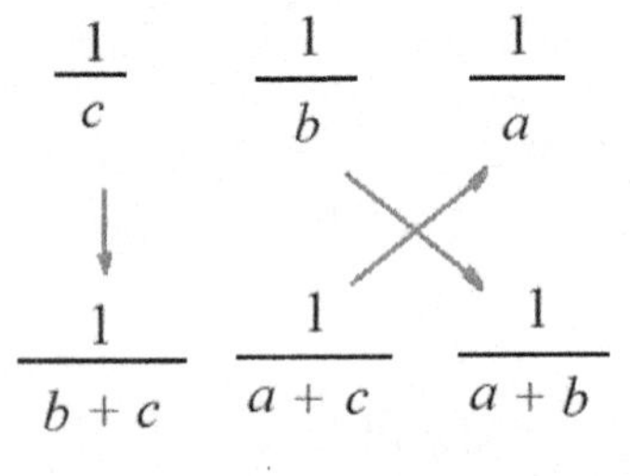

$\frac{1}{c} \quad \frac{1}{b} \quad \frac{1}{a}$

$\downarrow \quad \times$

$\frac{1}{b+c} \quad \frac{1}{a+c} \quad \frac{1}{a+b}$

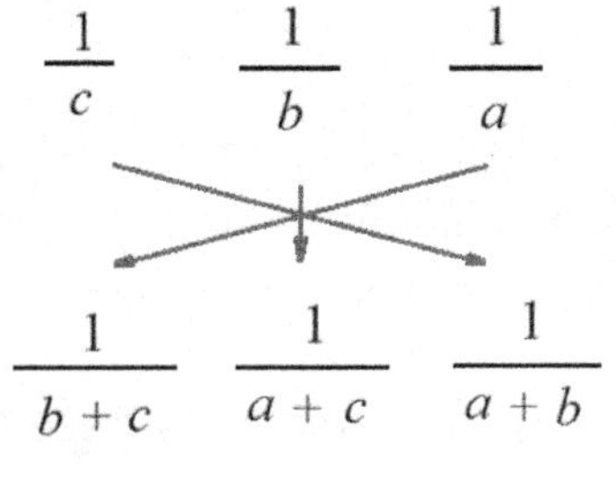

$\frac{1}{c} \quad \frac{1}{b} \quad \frac{1}{a}$

$\times$

$\frac{1}{b+c} \quad \frac{1}{a+c} \quad \frac{1}{a+b}$

$$\frac{1}{c(b+c)}+\frac{1}{b(a+b)}+\frac{1}{a(a+c)}\geq\frac{1}{c(a+b)}+\frac{1}{b(a+c)}+\frac{1}{a(b+c)}.$$

For case 2, $a \le c \le b$,
$\frac{1}{b} \le \frac{1}{c} \le \frac{1}{a}$. $\frac{1}{b+c} \le \frac{1}{a+b} \le \frac{1}{a+c}$.

For the two similarly sorted sequences
$\frac{1}{b}, \frac{1}{c}, \frac{1}{a}$
$\frac{1}{b+c}, \frac{1}{a+b}, \frac{1}{a+c}$
by the rearrangement inequality, we have

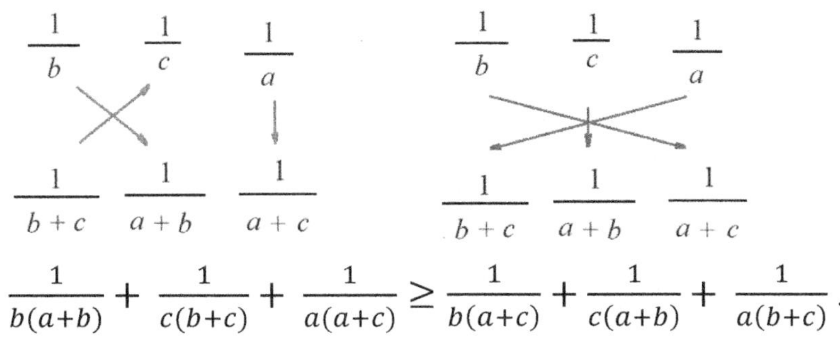

$$\frac{1}{b(a+b)}+\frac{1}{c(b+c)}+\frac{1}{a(a+c)}\geq\frac{1}{b(a+c)}+\frac{1}{c(a+b)}+\frac{1}{a(b+c)}.$$

Example 11. (1999 Canadian Math Olympiad) Let a, b, and c be non-negative real numbers satisfying $a + b + c = 1$. Show that $a^2b + b^2c + c^2a \le 4/27$, and find when equality occurs.

Solution:
Method 1:
The expression $a^2b + b^2c + c^2a$ is cyclic but not symmetric. WLOG, we may assume that $a = \min(a, b, c)$. Then we have two cases:
Case 1: $a \le b \le c$
Case 2: $a \le c \le b$.

For the first case, we get the following similarly ordered sequences,
a, b, c

ab, ac, bc

By the rearrangement inequality,

$$\begin{array}{cccccc} a & b & c & a & b & c \\ \downarrow & \multicolumn{2}{c}{\times} & \downarrow & \downarrow & \downarrow \\ ab & ac & bc & ab & ac & bc \end{array}$$

$a^2b + b^2c + c^2a \le a^2b + abc + c^2b = b(a^2 + ac + c^2)$

$\le b(a+c)^2 = \frac{1}{2}(2b)(a+c)(a+c) \le \frac{1}{2}(\frac{2b+(a+c)+(a+c)}{3})^3 = \frac{1}{2}(\frac{2}{3})^3 = \frac{4}{27}$,

where the last inequality follows from AM-GM inequality. Equality occurs if and only if $c = 0$ (from the first inequality) and $b = 1/3$, in which case $(a, b, c) = (\frac{2}{3}, \frac{1}{3}, 0)$.

For the second case, we can prove in a similar way.

Method 2 (official solution):

Let $f(x, y, z) = x^2y + y^2z + z^2x$.

We wish to determine where f is maximal. Since f is cyclic, WLOG, we may assume that $x \ge y, z$.

Since

$f(x, y, z) - f(x, z, y) = x^2y + y^2z + z^2x - x^2z - z^2y - y^2x = (y - z)(x - y)(x - z)$.

we may also assume $y \ge z$. Then

$f(x + z, y, 0) - f(x, z, y) = (x + z)^2y - x^2y - y^2z - z^2x = z^2y + yz(x - y) + xz(y - z) \ge 0$, so we may assume $z = 0$.

The rest follows from the arithmetic-geometric mean inequality:

$f(x, y, 0) = \frac{2x^2y}{2} \le \frac{1}{2}(\frac{x+x+2y}{3})^3 = \frac{4}{27}$.

Equality occurs when $x = 2y$, hence at $(x, z, y) = (\frac{2}{3}, \frac{1}{3}, 0)$. As well as $(0, \frac{2}{3}, \frac{1}{3})$ and $(\frac{1}{3}, 0, \frac{2}{3})$.

Example 12. (1983 IMO) Suppose that a, b, c are the side-lengths of a triangle. Prove that $a^2b(a-b)+b^2c(b-c)+c^2a(c-a)\ge 0$. Determine when equality occurs.

Solution:

Method 1:

The inequality is cyclic.

Consider the case $a\le b\le c$ (the other cases are similar). So we have $\frac{1}{c}\le\frac{1}{b}\le\frac{1}{a}$.

Thus $a^2+bc\le b^2+ca\le c^2+ab$.

Then we have the following two similarly ordered sequences:

$a^2+bc,\ b^2+ca,\ c^2+ab$.

$\frac{1}{c},\frac{1}{b},\frac{1}{a}$.

By the rearrangement inequality,

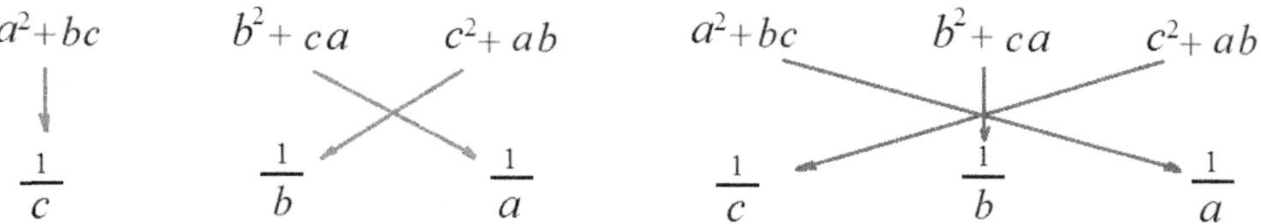

$$\frac{a^2+bc}{c}+\frac{b^2+ca}{a}+\frac{c^2+ab}{b}\ge\frac{a^2+bc}{a}+\frac{b^2+ca}{b}+\frac{c^2+ab}{c}$$

$$\Leftrightarrow \frac{a^2}{c}+b+\frac{b^2}{a}+c+\frac{c^2}{b}+a\ge a+\frac{bc}{a}+b+\frac{ca}{b}+c+\frac{c^2}{c}$$

$$\Leftrightarrow \frac{a^2}{c}+\frac{b^2}{a}+\frac{c^2}{b}\ge\frac{bc}{a}+\frac{ca}{b}+\frac{c^2}{c}$$

$$\Leftrightarrow \frac{a^2}{c}-\frac{c^2}{c}+\frac{b^2}{a}-\frac{bc}{a}+\frac{c^2}{b}-\frac{bc}{a}\ge 0$$

$$\Leftrightarrow a^2b(a-b)+b^2c(b-c)+c^2a(c-a)\ge 0.$$

Equality holds for $a=b=c$.

Method 2:

Let $a = y + z$, $b = z + x$, $c = x + y$. Then the triangle condition becomes simply x, y, $z > 0$. The inequality becomes (after some manipulation):
$xy^3 + yz^3 + zx^3 \geq xyz(x + y + z)$.
Dividing both sides by xyz, we have
$\frac{x^2}{y} + \frac{y^2}{z} + \frac{z^2}{x} \geq x + y + z$

The expression is not a symmetric function of x, y and z. However, we have the following similarly ordered sequences:
x^2, y^2, z^2
$\frac{1}{z}, \frac{1}{y}, \frac{1}{x}$.

By the rearrangement inequality,

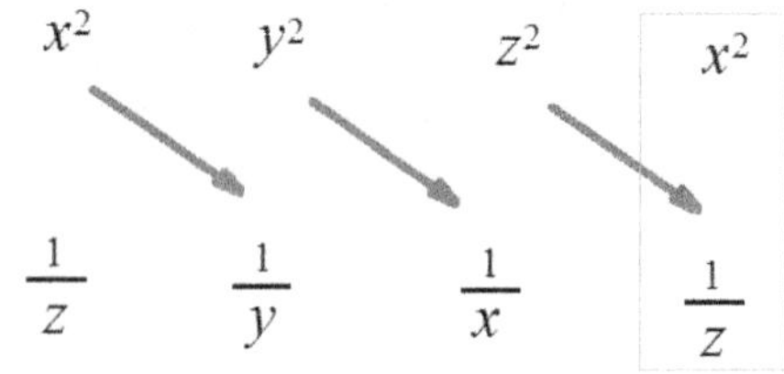

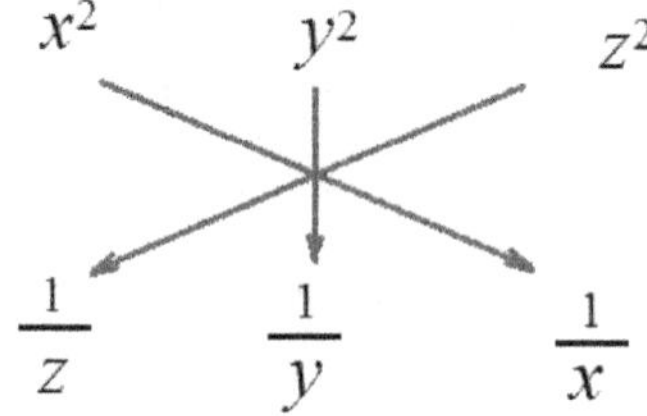

$$\frac{x^2}{y} + \frac{y^2}{z} + \frac{z^2}{x} \geq \frac{x^2}{x} + \frac{y^2}{y} + \frac{z^2}{z} = x + y + z$$
with equality $x^2 = y^2 = z^2$ or $\frac{1}{z} = \frac{1}{y} = \frac{1}{x}$.
Thus the original inequality holds with equality iff the triangle is equilateral.

Method 3:
We may assume $a \leq b \leq c$, we first prove that $a(b + c - a) \geq b(c + a - b) \geq c(a + b - c)$. Note that $b(c + a - b) - a(b + c - a) = (a - b)(a + b - c) \leq 0$. The second inequality reduces to $(b - c)(b + c - a) \leq 0$ and is obvious by the triangle inequality.
Dividing the given inequality by abc we have to show that
$\frac{1}{c}a(a - b) + \frac{1}{a}b(b - c) + \frac{1}{b}c(c - a) \geq 0$ or after subtracting $a + b + c$, that

$\frac{1}{c}a(-c+a-b)+\frac{1}{a}b(-a+b-c)+\frac{1}{b}c(-b+c-a)\geq-(a+b+c)$.

The desire inequality can be written as

$\frac{1}{c}a(c-a+b)+\frac{1}{a}b(a-b+c)+\frac{1}{b}c(b-c+a)\leq a+b+c$.

Then we have the following two similarly ordered sequences:

$a(c-a+b),(a-b+c),c(b-c+a)$

$\frac{1}{c},\frac{1}{b},\frac{1}{a}$

By the rearrangement inequality

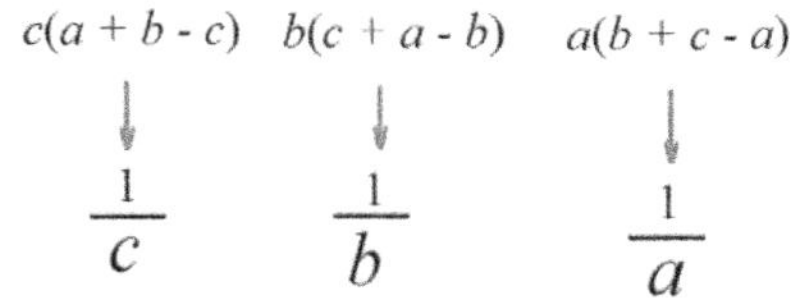

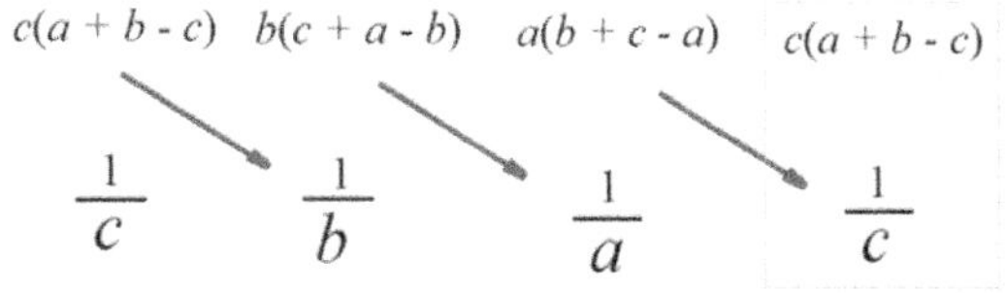

$c(a+b-c)$ $b(c+a-b)$ $a(b+c-a)$ $c(a+b-c)$ $b(c+a-b)$ $a(b+c-a)$ $c(a+b-c)$

$\frac{1}{c}$ $\frac{1}{b}$ $\frac{1}{a}$ $\frac{1}{c}$ $\frac{1}{b}$ $\frac{1}{a}$ $\frac{1}{c}$

$$\frac{1}{c}c(a+b-c)+\frac{1}{b}b(c+a-b)+\frac{1}{a}a(b+c-a)=a+b+c$$

$\geq\frac{1}{c}a(c-a+b)+\frac{1}{a}b(a-b+c)+\frac{1}{b}c(b-c+a)$. QED.

CHAPTER 5. PROBLEMS

Problem 1. Is the expression $\frac{ab}{c}+\frac{cb}{a}+\frac{ac}{b}$ cyclic?

Problem 2. Is the expression $\frac{a^2}{a+1}+\frac{b^2}{b+1}$ cyclic?

Problem 3. Is the expression $\frac{ab}{c(b+c)}+\frac{bc}{a(c+a)}+\frac{ca}{b(a+b)}$ cyclic?

Problem 4. Is the inequality $\frac{a^2}{b^2}+\frac{b^2}{c^2}+\frac{c^2}{a^2}\geq a^2+b^2+c^2$ cyclic?

Problem 5. Is the expression cyclic?
$\frac{a^2+c^2}{b}+\frac{b^2+a^2}{c}+\frac{c^2+a^2}{a}$

Problem 6. Is the expression $\frac{a}{\sqrt{b+c}}+\frac{b}{\sqrt{c+a}}+\frac{c}{\sqrt{a+b}}$ cyclic?

Problem 7. Prove that for all positive real numbers, $\frac{a^2b}{c}+\frac{b^2c}{a}+\frac{c^2a}{b}\geq ab+bc+ca$.

Problem 8. For nonnegative numbers a, b, c, if $a+b+c=3$, prove that $(a^2b+b^2c+c^2a)(ab+bc+ca)\leq 9$.

Problem 9. (Middle European Mathematical Olympiad 2007) Let a, b, c, d be non-negative real numbers such that $a+b+c+d=4$. Prove that $a^2bc+b^2cd+c^2da+d^2ab\leq 4$.

Problem 10. Let a, b, c be real numbers. Prove the inequality
$a^5+b^5+c^5\geq abc(a^2+b^2+c^2)$.

Problem 11. Show that $a\sqrt{\frac{1+a^2}{1+b^2}} + b\sqrt{\frac{1+b^2}{1+c^2}} + c\sqrt{\frac{1+c^2}{1+a^2}} \geq a+b+c$. a, b, c are positive real numbers.

Problem 12. Let *a, b*, and *c* be positive real numbers. Prove that

$$\left(\frac{5a-b}{b+c}\right)^2 + \left(\frac{5b-c}{c+a}\right)^2 + \left(\frac{5c-a}{a+b}\right)^2 \geq 12.$$

CHAPTER 5. SOLUTIONS

Problem 1. Solution: Yes.

If we change *a* for *b*, *b* for *c*, and *c* for *a*, we have $\frac{bc}{a}+\frac{ac}{b}+\frac{ba}{c}$ which is the same as the given expression. So this expression is cyclic.

Problem 2. Solution: Yes.

If we change *a* for *b*, we have $\frac{b^2}{b+1}+\frac{a^2}{a+1}$ which is the same as the given expression. So this expression is cyclic.

Problem 3. Solution: Yes.

If we change *a* for *b*, *b* for *c*, and *c* for *a*, we have $\frac{ab}{c(b+c)}+\frac{bc}{a(c+a)}+\frac{ca}{b(a+b)}$ which is the same as the given expression. So this expression is cyclic.

Problem 4. Solution: Yes.

If we change *a* for *b*, *b* for *c*, and *c* for *a*, we have $\frac{a^2}{b^2}+\frac{b^2}{c^2}+\frac{c^2}{a^2}\geq a^2+b^2+c^2$.

which is the same as the given expression. So this expression is cyclic.

Problem 5. Solution: No.

We do the following replacements:

$a \Rightarrow b \Rightarrow c$, and we get

$\frac{b^2+a^2}{c}+\frac{c^2+b^2}{a}+\frac{a^2+b^2}{b}$.

We see that the new expression is different from the given one. So it is not cyclic.

Problem 6. Solution: Yes.

If we change *a* for *b*, *b* for *c*, and *c* for *a*, we have $\frac{b}{\sqrt{c+a}}+\frac{c}{\sqrt{a+b}}+\frac{a}{\sqrt{b+c}}$ which is the same as the given expression. So this expression is cyclic.

Problem 7. Solution:

We see that the given inequality is cyclic. Let us assume that

Case 1: $a \le b \le c$.

Case 2: $a \le c \le b$.

For case 1, since $a \le b \le c$, we know that $ab \le ac \le bc$,

$\frac{ab}{c} \le \frac{ac}{b} \le \frac{bc}{a}$

Then we have the following two similarly ordered sequences:

$a, b, c,$

$\frac{ab}{c}, \frac{ac}{b}, \frac{bc}{a}.$

By the rearrangement inequality, we have

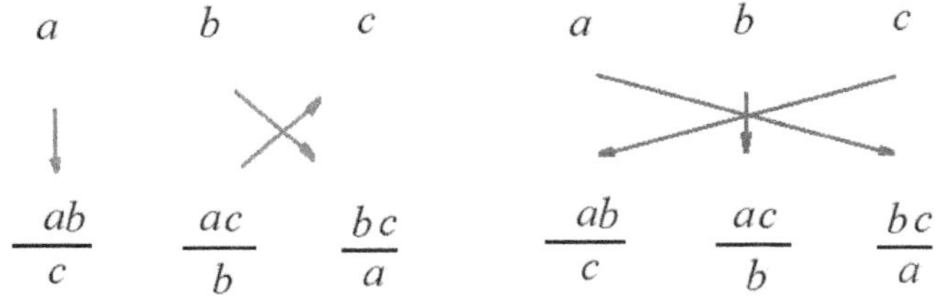

$$\frac{a^2b}{c} + \frac{b^2c}{a} + \frac{c^2a}{b} \ge a\cdot\frac{bc}{a} + b\cdot\frac{ac}{b} + c\cdot\frac{ab}{c} = bc + ac + ab\ .$$

The case 2 can be dealt similarly.

Problem 8. Solution:

The expression $(a^2b + b^2c + c^2a)(ab + bc + ca)$ is cyclic but not symmetric. WLOG, we may assume that $a = \min(a, b, c)$. Then we have two cases:

Case 1: $a \le b \le c$

Case 2: $a \le c \le b$.

For the first case, we get the following similarly ordered sequences,

a, b, c

ab, ac, bc

By the rearrangement inequality, we have

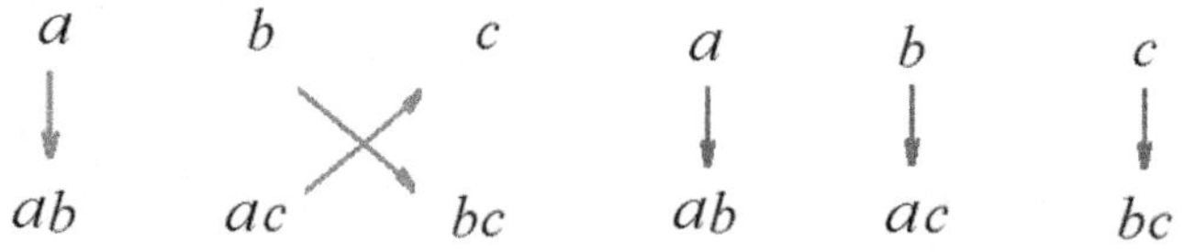

$a \quad b \quad c \qquad a \quad b \quad c$

$ab \quad ac \quad bc \qquad ab \quad ac \quad bc$

$$a^2b + b^2c + c^2a \le a^2b + abc + c^2b = b(a^2 + ac + c^2) \qquad (1)$$

$(1) \times (ab + bc + ca)$:

$$(ab + bc + ca)(a^2b + b^2c + c^2a) \le (ab + bc + ca)\, b(a^2 + ac + c^2)$$

$$= b \cdot \frac{(ab + bc + ca)b(a^2 + ac + c^2)^2}{4} = b \cdot \frac{(ab + bc + ca)\, b(a^2 + ac + c^2)^2}{4}$$

$$= b \cdot \frac{(a+c)^2(a+b+c)^2}{4} = \frac{9b(a+c)^2}{4} = \frac{9}{8}(2b)(a+c)(a+c) \le \frac{9}{8}\left(\frac{2(a+b+c)}{3}\right)^3 = 9.$$

For the second case, we prove in a similar way.

Problem 9. Solution:

Method 1:

Since the expression is a not symmetric but cyclic of a, b and c, we can assume, without loss of generality, that $a = \min\{a, b, c, d)$ and $d = \max\{a, b, c, d)$. Thus we have two cases: (1) $a \le b \le c \le d$, $abc \le abd \le acd \le bcd$.

(2) $a \le c \le b \le d$, $abc \le acd \le abd \le bcd$.

For case 1, we have the following two similarly ordered sequences:

$a,\ b,\ c,\ d$

$abc,\ abd,\ acd,\ bcd.$

By the rearrangement inequality, we have

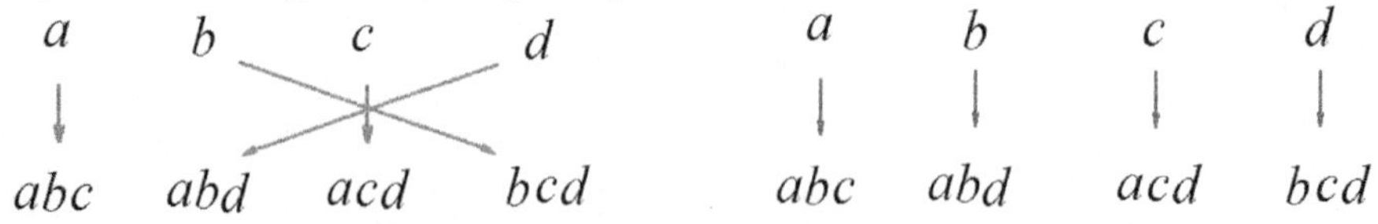

$a \quad b \quad c \quad d \qquad a \quad b \quad c \quad d$

$abc \quad abd \quad acd \quad bcd \qquad abc \quad abd \quad acd \quad bcd$

$$a^2bc + b^2cd + c^2ad + d^2ab$$

$$\le a^2bc + b^2ad + c^2ad + d^2bc$$

$$= (ab + cd)(ac + bd)$$

$$\le \left(\frac{ab+ac+bd+cd}{2}\right)^2 \le \frac{1}{4}(ab + ac + bd + cd)^2 = \frac{1}{4}(a+c)^2(b+d)^2$$

$\leq \frac{1}{4}[(\frac{a+c+b+d}{2})^2]^2 = \frac{16}{4} = 4$

Equality holds for $a = b = c = d = 1$
or $a = 2$, $b = c = 1$, $d = 0$ up to permutation.

We can prove the case 2 in a similar way.

Method 2:
Suppose that (x, y, z, t) is a permutation of (a, b, c, d) such that $x \leq y \leq z \leq t$, then $xyz \leq xyt \leq axzt \leq yzt$.

By Rearrangement inequality, we deduce that
$x \cdot xyz + y.\ xyt + z \cdot xzt + t \cdot yzt \geq a^2bc + b^2cd + c^2da + d^2ab.$

According to AM-GM inequality, we also have

$x \cdot xyz + y.\ xyt + z \cdot xzt + t \cdot yzt = (xy + zt)(xz + yt) \leq \frac{1}{4}(xy + xz + yt + zt)^2 \leq 4.$

Thus $a^2bc + b^2cd + c^2da + d^2ab \leq 4$.
Equality holds for
$a = b = c = d = 1$ or $a = 2$, $b = c = 1$, $d = 0$ up to permutation.

Problem 10. Solution:
Without loss of generality we may assume that $a \leq b \leq c$, and then clearly $a^3 \leq b^3 \leq c^3$.

Now by the rearrangement inequality, we get the required inequality.

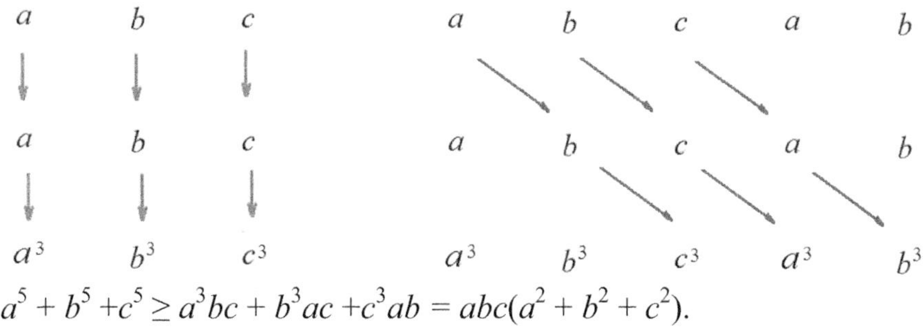

$a^5 + b^5 + c^5 \geq a^3bc + b^3ac + c^3ab = abc(a^2 + b^2 + c^2).$

Problem 11. Proof:

The given expression is not symmetric but cyclic. So we are not able to assume that $a \le b \le c$. However, we can, WLOG, assume that a is $\min\{a, b, c\}$. Thus we have two cases: 1: $a \le b \le c$, and 2: $a \le c \le b$.

For case 1, $a \le b \le c$, $\sqrt{1+a^2} \le \sqrt{1+b^2} \le \sqrt{1+c^2}$, $a\sqrt{1+a^2} \le b\sqrt{1+b^2} \le c\sqrt{1+c^2}$, $\frac{1}{\sqrt{1+c^2}} \le \frac{1}{\sqrt{1+b^2}} \le \frac{1}{\sqrt{1+a^2}}$.

For the two similarly sorted sequences

$a\sqrt{1+a^2}, b\sqrt{1+b^2}, c\sqrt{1+c^2}$

$\frac{1}{\sqrt{1+c^2}}, \frac{1}{\sqrt{1+b^2}}, \frac{1}{\sqrt{1+a^2}}$,

by the rearrangement inequality, we have

$a\sqrt{1+a^2} \quad b\sqrt{1+b^2} \quad c\sqrt{1+c^2}$ $\qquad$ $a\sqrt{1+a^2} \quad b\sqrt{1+b^2} \quad c\sqrt{1+c^2}$

$\frac{1}{\sqrt{1+c^2}} \quad \frac{1}{\sqrt{1+b^2}} \quad \frac{1}{\sqrt{1+a^2}}$ $\qquad$ $\frac{1}{\sqrt{1+c^2}} \quad \frac{1}{\sqrt{1+b^2}} \quad \frac{1}{\sqrt{1+a^2}}$

$$a\sqrt{1+a^2} \cdot \frac{1}{\sqrt{1+b^2}} + b\sqrt{1+b^2} \cdot \frac{1}{\sqrt{1+c^2}} + c\sqrt{1+c^2} \cdot \frac{1}{\sqrt{1+a^2}} \ge a\sqrt{1+a^2} \cdot \frac{1}{\sqrt{1+a^2}} + b\sqrt{1+b^2} \cdot \frac{1}{\sqrt{1+b^2}} + c\sqrt{1+c^2} \cdot \frac{1}{\sqrt{1+c^2}} = a + b + c.$$

For case 2, $a \le c \le b$, $\sqrt{1+a^2} \le \sqrt{1+c^2} \le \sqrt{1+b^2}$, $a\sqrt{1+a^2} \le c\sqrt{1+c^2} \le b\sqrt{1+b^2}$, $\frac{1}{\sqrt{1+b^2}} \le \frac{1}{\sqrt{1+c^2}} \le \frac{1}{\sqrt{1+a^2}}$.

For the two similarly sorted sequences

$a\sqrt{1+a^2}, c\sqrt{1+c^2}, b\sqrt{1+b^2}$

$\frac{1}{\sqrt{1+b^2}}, \frac{1}{\sqrt{1+c^2}}, \frac{1}{\sqrt{1+a^2}}$

by the rearrangement inequality, we have

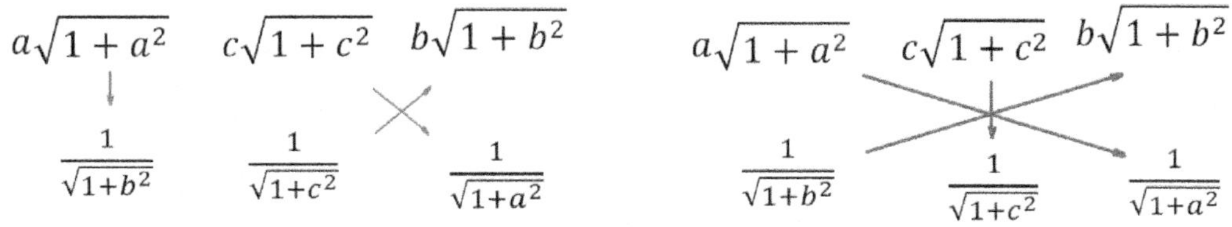

$a\sqrt{1+a^2}$ $c\sqrt{1+c^2}$ $b\sqrt{1+b^2}$ $a\sqrt{1+a^2}$ $c\sqrt{1+c^2}$ $b\sqrt{1+b^2}$

$\frac{1}{\sqrt{1+b^2}}$ $\frac{1}{\sqrt{1+c^2}}$ $\frac{1}{\sqrt{1+a^2}}$ $\frac{1}{\sqrt{1+b^2}}$ $\frac{1}{\sqrt{1+c^2}}$ $\frac{1}{\sqrt{1+a^2}}$

$a\sqrt{1+a^2}\cdot\frac{1}{\sqrt{1+b^2}}+b\sqrt{1+b^2}\cdot\frac{1}{\sqrt{1+c^2}}+c\sqrt{1+c^2}\cdot\frac{1}{\sqrt{1+a^2}}\geq a\sqrt{1+a^2}\cdot\frac{1}{\sqrt{1+a^2}}+$
$b\sqrt{1+b^2}\cdot\frac{1}{\sqrt{1+b^2}}+c\sqrt{1+c^2}\cdot\frac{1}{\sqrt{1+c^2}}=a+b+c.$

Problem 12. Solution.
Solution:

$$\left(\frac{5a-b}{b+c}\right)^2+\left(\frac{5b-c}{c+a}\right)^2+\left(\frac{5c-a}{a+b}\right)^2\geq 12 \quad (1)$$

The given expression is not symmetric but cyclic. So we are not able to assume that $a \leq b \leq c$. However, we can, WLOG, assume that a is $\min\{a, b, c\}$. Thus we have two cases: 1: $a \leq b \leq c$, and 2: $a \leq c \leq b$.

For case 1, since $b + c \geq a + c \geq a + b$, we have the following two similarly ordered sequences:

c, b, a

$\frac{1}{b+c}, \frac{1}{a+c}, \frac{1}{a+b}$

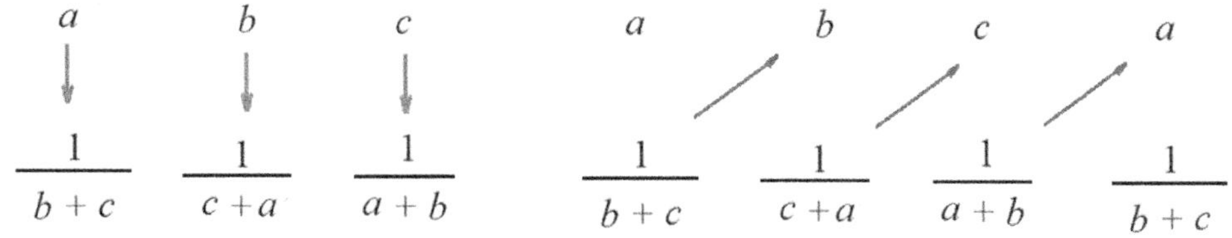

a b c a b c a

$\frac{1}{b+c}$ $\frac{1}{c+a}$ $\frac{1}{a+b}$ $\frac{1}{b+c}$ $\frac{1}{c+a}$ $\frac{1}{a+b}$ $\frac{1}{b+c}$

$$2\left(\frac{a}{b+c}+\frac{b}{c+a}+\frac{c}{a+b}\right)\geq 2\left(\frac{b}{b+c}+\frac{c}{c+a}+\frac{a}{a+b}\right) \quad (2)$$

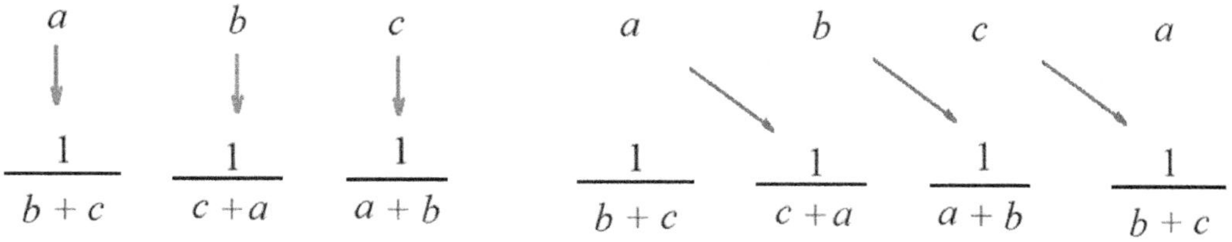

a b c a b c a

$\frac{1}{b+c}$ $\frac{1}{c+a}$ $\frac{1}{a+b}$ $\frac{1}{b+c}$ $\frac{1}{c+a}$ $\frac{1}{a+b}$ $\frac{1}{b+c}$

$$2(\frac{a}{b+c}+\frac{b}{c+a}+\frac{c}{a+b}) \geq 2(\frac{c}{b+c}+\frac{a}{c+a}+\frac{b}{a+b}) \qquad (3)$$

$$\frac{a}{b+c}+\frac{b}{c+a}+\frac{c}{a+b} \geq \frac{b}{b+c}+\frac{c}{c+a}+\frac{a}{a+b} \qquad (4)$$

(1) + (2) + (3):

$$5\left(\frac{a}{b+c}+\frac{b}{c+a}+\frac{c}{a+b}\right) \geq 6+\frac{b}{b+c}+\frac{c}{c+a}+\frac{a}{a+b}$$

From which we obtain

$$\frac{5a-b}{b+c}+\frac{5b-c}{c+a}+\frac{5c-a}{a+b} \geq 6 \qquad (5)$$

We write (5) as $x+y+z \geq 6$ (6)

and (1) $x^2+y^2+z^2 \geq 12$ (7)

From (6), $(x+y+z)^2 \geq 36 \quad \Rightarrow \quad x^2+y^2+z^2+2(xy+yz+zx) \geq 36$

$\Rightarrow \quad x^2+y^2+z^2 \geq 36-2(xy+yz+zx)$

$\Rightarrow \quad x^2+y^2+z^2 \geq 36-2(x^2+y^2+z^2)$

$\Rightarrow \quad 3(x^2+y^2+z^2) \geq 36$

$\Rightarrow \quad x^2+y^2+z^2 \geq 12.$

So we have proved ((7).

For case 2, we prove in a similar way. QED.

Chapter 6. Rearrangement With AM-GM And Cauchy Combined

General Form of the *AM-GM* Inequality

In general, for nonnegative real numbers $a_1, a_2, \ldots a_n$,

the arithmetic mean of n numbers is: $A_n = \dfrac{a_1 + a_2 + \ldots + a_n}{n}$

the geometric mean of n numbers is: $G_n = (a_1 \times a_2 \times \ldots \times a_n)^{\frac{1}{n}} = \sqrt[n]{a_1 \times a_2 \times \ldots \times a_n}$.

We have the following relationship between the arithmetic mean and the geometric mean:

$$\frac{a_1 + a_2 + \ldots + a_n}{n} \geq \sqrt[n]{a_1 \times a_2 \times \ldots \times a_n}$$

or $a_1 + a_2 + \ldots + a_n \geq n\sqrt[n]{a_1 \times a_2 \times \ldots \times a_n}$

Equality occurs if and only if $a_1 = a_2 = \ldots = a_n$.

For three terms, $\dfrac{a+b+c}{3} \geq \sqrt[3]{abc}$, or $a+b+c \geq 3\sqrt[3]{abc}$, or $abc \leq (\dfrac{a+b+c}{3})^3$.

Cauchy's Inequality

Let $a_1, a_2, a_3, \ldots, a_n$, and $b_1, b_2, b_3, \ldots, b_n$ be real numbers. Then

$$(a_1^2 + a_2^2 + \ldots + a_n^2) \cdot (b_1^2 + b_2^2 + \ldots + b_n^2) \geq (a_1 b_1 + a_2 b_2 + \ldots + a_n b_n)^2$$

Equality occurs if and only if $b_i = 0 (i = 1, 2, \ldots, n)$ or $a_i = k b_i (i = 1, 2, \ldots, n)$.

Cauchy's Inequality in Three Terms:

Let a_1, a_2, a_3, and b_1, b_2, b_3 be real numbers. Then

$$(a_1^2 + a_2^2 + a_3^2) \cdot (b_1^2 + b_2^2 + b_3^2) \geq (a_1 b_1 + a_2 b_2 + a_3 b_3)^2$$

Equality occurs if and only if $b_i = 0 (i = 1, 2, 3)$ or $a_i = kb_i (i = 1, 2, 3)$.

Different form of Cauchy's Inequality in Three Terms:

If a, b are real numbers and x, y are positive numbers then

$$\frac{a^2}{x} + \frac{b^2}{y} + \frac{c^2}{z} \geq \frac{(a+b+c)^2}{x+y+z}$$

Equality occurs if and only if $\frac{a}{x} = \frac{b}{y} = \frac{c}{z}$.

Example 1. For nonnegative numbers a, b, c, with $abc = 1$, show that $a^3 + b^3 + c^3 \geq a^2 + b^2 + c^2$.

Proof:

Method 1:

We have the following similarly ordered sequences,

$a,\ b,\ c$

$a^2, b^2\ c^2$

By the rearrangement inequality, we have

$$a^3 + b^3 + c^3 \geq a^3 + b^3 + c^3 \qquad (1)$$

$$\begin{matrix} a & b & c \\ \downarrow & \downarrow & \downarrow \\ a^2 & b^2 & c^2 \end{matrix} \qquad \begin{matrix} a & & b & & c & & a \\ & \searrow & & \searrow & & \searrow & \\ a^2 & & b^2 & & c^2 & & a^2 \end{matrix}$$

or $\begin{bmatrix} a & b & c \\ a^2 & b^2 & c^2 \end{bmatrix} \geq \begin{bmatrix} a & b & c \\ b^2 & c^2 & a^2 \end{bmatrix}$

$$a^3 + b^3 + c^3 \geq ab^2 + bc^2 + ca^2 \qquad (2)$$

$$\begin{matrix} a & b & c \\ \downarrow & \downarrow & \downarrow \\ a^2 & b^2 & c^2 \end{matrix} \qquad \begin{matrix} a & & b & & c & & a \\ & \nearrow & & \nearrow & & \nearrow & \\ a^2 & & b^2 & & c^2 & & a^2 \end{matrix}$$

or $\begin{bmatrix} a & b & c \\ a^2 & b^2 & c^2 \end{bmatrix} \geq \begin{bmatrix} a & b & c \\ c^2 & a^2 & b^2 \end{bmatrix}$

$$a^3 + b^3 + c^3 \geq ac^2 + ba^2 + cb^2 \qquad (3)$$

(1) + (2) + (3):

$3(a^3 + b^3 + c^3) \geq a^3 + b^3 + c^3 + ab^2 + bc^2 + ca^2 + a^2b + b^2c + c^2a$

$= (a^3 + ab^2 + c^2a) + (b^3 + bc^2 + a^2b) + (c^3 + b^2c + ca^2)$

$= a(a^2 + b^2 + c^2) + b(b^2 + c^2 + a^2) + c(c^2 + b^2 + a^2)$

$= (a + b + c)(a^2 + b^2 + c^2)$

$\geq 3\sqrt[3]{abc}\,(a^2 + b^2 + c^2) = 3(a^2 + b^2 + c^2).$

Thus $a^3 + b^3 + c^3 \geq a^2 + b^2 + c^2$. QED.

Note: for any positive integer n, with $abc = 1$: $3 \leq a + b + c \leq a^2 + b^2 + c^2 \leq a^3 + b^3 + c^3 \leq a^4 + b^4 + c^4 \leq \ldots \leq a^n + b^n + c^n$.

Method 2:

Since $abc = 1$, we have $\sqrt[3]{abc} = \sqrt[3]{a} \cdot \sqrt[3]{b} \cdot \sqrt[3]{c} = 1$.

We have the following similarly ordered sequences,

$\sqrt[3]{a}, \sqrt[3]{b}, \sqrt[3]{c}$

$\sqrt[3]{a}, \sqrt[3]{b}, \sqrt[3]{c}$

$\sqrt[3]{a^7}, \sqrt[3]{b^7}, \sqrt[3]{c^7},$

By the rearrangement inequality, we have

$$\begin{matrix} \sqrt[3]{a} & \sqrt[3]{b} & \sqrt[3]{a} \\ \downarrow & \downarrow & \downarrow \\ \sqrt[3]{a} & \sqrt[3]{b} & \sqrt[3]{a} \\ \downarrow & \downarrow & \downarrow \\ \sqrt[3]{a^7} & \sqrt[3]{b^7} & \sqrt[3]{c^7} \end{matrix} \qquad \begin{matrix} \sqrt[3]{a} & \sqrt[3]{b} & \sqrt[3]{c} & \sqrt[3]{a} & \sqrt[3]{b} \\ \sqrt[3]{a} & \sqrt[3]{b} & \sqrt[3]{c} & \sqrt[3]{a} & \sqrt[3]{b} \\ \sqrt[3]{a^7} & \sqrt[3]{b^7} & \sqrt[3]{c^7} & \sqrt[3]{a^7} & \sqrt[3]{b^7} \end{matrix}$$

$$\text{or}\begin{bmatrix} \sqrt[3]{a} & \sqrt[3]{b} & \sqrt[3]{c} \\ \sqrt[3]{a} & \sqrt[3]{b} & \sqrt[3]{c} \\ \sqrt[3]{a^7} & \sqrt[3]{b^7} & \sqrt[3]{c^7} \end{bmatrix} \geq \begin{bmatrix} \sqrt[3]{a} & \sqrt[3]{b} & \sqrt[3]{c} \\ \sqrt[3]{b} & \sqrt[3]{c} & \sqrt[3]{a} \\ \sqrt[3]{c^7} & \sqrt[3]{a^7} & \sqrt[3]{b^7} \end{bmatrix}$$

$\sqrt[3]{a}\cdot\sqrt[3]{a}\cdot\sqrt[3]{a^7}+\sqrt[3]{b}\cdot\sqrt[3]{b}\cdot\sqrt[3]{b^7}+\sqrt[3]{c}\cdot\sqrt[3]{c}\cdot\sqrt[3]{c^7}$
$\geq \sqrt[3]{a}\cdot\sqrt[3]{b}\cdot\sqrt[3]{c^7}+\sqrt[3]{b}\cdot\sqrt[3]{c}\cdot\sqrt[3]{a^7}+\sqrt[3]{c}\cdot\sqrt[3]{a}\cdot\sqrt[3]{b^7} \qquad \Rightarrow$
$\sqrt[3]{a^9}+\sqrt[3]{b^9}+\sqrt[3]{c^9} \geq \sqrt[3]{a}\cdot\sqrt[3]{b}\cdot\sqrt[3]{c}\cdot\sqrt[3]{c^6}+\sqrt[3]{b}\cdot\sqrt[3]{c}\cdot\sqrt[3]{a}\cdot\sqrt[3]{a^6}+\sqrt[3]{c}\cdot\sqrt[3]{a}\cdot\sqrt[3]{b}\cdot$
$\sqrt[3]{b^6}$
Thus $a^3+b^3+c^3 \geq a^2+b^2+c^2$. QED.

Example 2. Suppose that a, b, c are positive real numbers such that $a \leq b \leq c$ and $a^2+b^2+c^2=3$, prove that $a^3b^2+b^3c^2+c^3a^2 \leq 3$.

Solution:
Since $a \leq b \leq c$, we have $a^2b^2 \leq a^2c^2 \leq b^2c^2$.

Then we have the following two similarly ordered sequences:
$a,\ b,\ c$
$a^2b^2,\ a^2c^2,\ b^2c^2$.

By the rearrangement inequality,

$$\begin{matrix} a & b & c \\ \downarrow & \times & \\ a^2b^2 & c^2a^2 & b^2c^2 \end{matrix} \qquad \begin{matrix} a & b & c \\ \downarrow & \downarrow & \downarrow \\ a^2b^2 & c^2a^2 & b^2c^2 \end{matrix}$$

$a\cdot a^2b^2+b\cdot b^2c^2+c\cdot c^2a^2 \leq a\cdot a^2b^2+b\cdot c^2a^2+c\cdot b^2c^2$
$= b(a^3b+c^2a^2+bc^3)$
$= b(a^3b+\frac{c^2a^2}{2}+bc^3+\frac{c^2a^2}{2})$
$= b[a^2\left(ab+\frac{c^2}{2}\right)+c^2\left(bc+\frac{a^2}{2}\right)]$
$\leq b[a^2\left(\frac{a^2+b^2+c^2}{2}\right)+c^2\left(\frac{a^2+b^2+c^2}{2}\right)]$

$= \frac{3}{2}b(a^2 + c^2) = \frac{3}{2}\sqrt{\frac{2b^2(a^2+c^2)(a^2+c^2)}{2}}$

$\le \frac{3}{2}\sqrt{\frac{(\frac{2b^2 + a^2 + c^2 + a^2 + c^2}{3})^3}{2}}$

$= \frac{3}{2}\sqrt{\frac{(2)^3}{2}} = 3$. QED.

Equality holds when $a = b = c = 1$.

Example 3. For nonnegative numbers a, b, c, $(a + b + c)(a^2 + b^2 + c^2) \ge 9abc$

Solution:
For the following similarly ordered sequences,

$a,\ \ b,\ \ c$

$a,\ \ b,\ \ c$

by the rearrangement inequality, we have

$$\begin{array}{ccc} a & b & c \\ \downarrow & \downarrow & \downarrow \\ a & b & c \end{array} \qquad \begin{array}{cccc} a & b & c & a \\ & \searrow & \searrow & \searrow \\ a & b & c & a \end{array}$$

$a^2 + b^2 + c^2 \ge ab + bc + ca$ (1)

$(1) \times (a + b + c)$:

$(a + b + c)(a^2 + b^2 + c^2) \ge (a + b + c)(ab + bc + ca)$

or $(a+b+c)\,(a^2 + b^2 + c^2) \ge 3\sqrt[3]{abc} \cdot 3\sqrt[3]{a^2b^2c^2} = 9abc$.

Example 4. (Russia, 1992) For any real numbers $a, b > 1$, prove that $\frac{a^2}{b-1} + \frac{b^2}{a-1} \ge 8$.

Solution:

Since the inequality is symmetric, WLOG, we may assume that $a \le b$. Then we know that $a^2 \le b^2$ and $\frac{1}{b-1} \le \frac{1}{a-1}$.

Then we have the following two similarly ordered sequences:
a^2, b^2
$\frac{1}{b-1}, \frac{1}{a-1}$

By the rearrangement inequality, we have

$$\begin{array}{cc} a^2 & b^2 \\ \downarrow & \downarrow \\ \frac{1}{b-1} & \frac{1}{a-1} \end{array} \qquad \begin{array}{cc} a^2 & b^2 \\ \multicolumn{2}{c}{\times} \\ \frac{1}{b-1} & \frac{1}{a-1} \end{array}$$

$$\frac{a^2}{b-1} + \frac{b^2}{a-1} \ge \frac{a^2}{a-1} + \frac{b^2}{b-1} = \frac{a^2-1+1}{a-1} + \frac{b^2-1+1}{b-1}$$

$$= a + 1 + \frac{1}{a-1} + b + 1 + \frac{1}{b-1}$$
$$= (a-1) + \left(\frac{1}{a-1}\right) + (b-1) + \left(\frac{1}{b-1}\right) + 4$$
$$\ge 2\sqrt{(a-1)\cdot\left(\frac{1}{a-1}\right)} + 2\sqrt{(b-1)\cdot\left(\frac{1}{b-1}\right)} + 4 = 2 + 2 + 4 = 8.$$

Example 5. Let *a, b, c* be positive real numbers. Prove that $\frac{a^3}{b^2} + \frac{b^3}{c^2} + \frac{c^3}{a^2} \ge \frac{a^2}{b} + \frac{b^2}{c} + \frac{c^2}{a}$.

Proof:
From AM-GM, we have

$$\frac{a^3}{b^2} + a \ge 2\sqrt{\frac{a^3}{b^2}\cdot a} = 2\frac{a^2}{b} \qquad (1)$$

Similarly,

$$\frac{b^3}{c^2}+b \geq 2\frac{b^2}{c} \qquad (2)$$

$$\frac{c^3}{a^2}+c \geq 2\frac{c^2}{a} \qquad (3)$$

(1) + (2) + (3):

$$\frac{a^3}{b^2}+\frac{b^3}{c^2}+\frac{c^3}{a^2}+a + b + c \geq 2(\frac{a^2}{b}+\frac{b^2}{c}+\frac{c^2}{a})$$

We have the following two similarly ordered sequences:

$a^2, b^2, c^2.$

$\frac{1}{c}, \frac{1}{b}, \frac{1}{a}$

By the rearrangement inequality, we have

$$\begin{array}{ccc} a^2 & b^2 & c^2 \\ \frac{1}{c} & \frac{1}{b} & \frac{1}{a} \end{array} \qquad \begin{array}{ccc} a^2 & b^2 & c^2 \\ \frac{1}{c} & \frac{1}{b} & \frac{1}{a} \end{array}$$

or $\begin{bmatrix} a^2 & b^2 & c^2 \\ \frac{1}{b} & \frac{1}{c} & \frac{1}{a} \end{bmatrix} \geq \begin{bmatrix} a^2 & b^2 & c^2 \\ \frac{1}{a} & \frac{1}{b} & \frac{1}{c} \end{bmatrix}$

Thus, $\frac{a^2}{b}+\frac{b^2}{c}+\frac{c^2}{a} \geq \frac{a^2}{a}+\frac{c^2}{c}+\frac{b^2}{b} = a+b+c$

Therefore,

$$\frac{a^3}{b^2}+\frac{b^3}{c^2}+\frac{c^3}{a^2}+a + b + c \geq \frac{a^2}{b}+\frac{b^2}{c}+\frac{c^2}{a}+a + b + c$$

That is $\frac{a^3}{b^2}+\frac{b^3}{c^2}+\frac{c^3}{a^2} \geq \frac{a^2}{b}+\frac{b^2}{c}+\frac{c^2}{a}$.

Example 6. Let a, b, $c > 0$ be real numbers. Prove the inequality $\frac{2a^2}{b+c}+\frac{2b^2}{c+a}+\frac{2c^2}{a+b}\geq a+b+c$.

Solution:

The given inequality can be written as

$$\frac{a^2}{b+c}+\frac{b^2}{c+a}+\frac{c^2}{a+b}\geq\frac{a+b+c}{2}$$

Since the expression is a symmetric function of a, b and c, we can assume, without loss of generality, that $a \leq b \leq c$. $a^2 \leq b^2 \leq c^2$. We also see that

$$\frac{1}{b+c}\leq\frac{1}{a+c}\leq\frac{1}{a+b}$$

Then we have the following two similarly ordered sequences:

$a^2,\ b^2,\ c^2$

$\frac{1}{b+c},\frac{1}{c+a},\frac{1}{a+b}$

By the rearrangement inequality, we have

$$\begin{array}{ccc} a^2 & b^2 & c^2 \\ \downarrow & \downarrow & \downarrow \\ \frac{1}{b+c} & \frac{1}{c+a} & \frac{1}{a+b} \end{array} \qquad \begin{array}{cccc} a^2 & b^2 & c^2 & a^2 \\ \searrow & \searrow & \searrow & \\ \frac{1}{b+c} & \frac{1}{c+a} & \frac{1}{a+b} & \frac{1}{b+c} \end{array}$$

$$\frac{a^2}{b+c}+\frac{b^2}{c+a}+\frac{c^2}{a+b}\geq\frac{a^2}{c+a}+\frac{b^2}{a+b}+\frac{c^2}{b+c} \qquad (1)$$

$$\begin{array}{ccc} a^2 & b^2 & c^2 \\ \downarrow & \downarrow & \downarrow \\ \frac{1}{b+c} & \frac{1}{c+a} & \frac{1}{a+b} \end{array} \qquad \begin{array}{cccc} a^2 & b^2 & c^2 & a^2 \\ \nearrow & \nearrow & \nearrow & \\ \frac{1}{b+c} & \frac{1}{c+a} & \frac{1}{a+b} & \frac{1}{b+c} \end{array}$$

$$\frac{a^2}{b+c}+\frac{b^2}{c+a}+\frac{c^2}{a+b}\geq\frac{b^2}{b+c}+\frac{c^2}{c+a}+\frac{a^2}{a+b} \qquad (2)$$

(1) + (2):

$$2\left(\frac{a^2}{b+c}+\frac{b^2}{c+a}+\frac{c^2}{a+b}\right)\geq\frac{a^2+c^2}{c+a}+\frac{b^2+a^2}{a+b}+\frac{c^2+b^2}{b+c} \qquad (3)$$

By Cauchy, $a^2+c^2=\frac{a^2}{1}+\frac{c^2}{1}\geq\frac{(a+c)^2}{2}$, $b^2+a^2\geq\frac{(b+a)^2}{2}$, $c^2+b^2\geq\frac{(c+b)^2}{2}$.
Substituting these values to (3):

$$2\left(\frac{a^2}{b+c}+\frac{b^2}{c+a}+\frac{c^2}{a+b}\right)\geq\frac{a+c}{2}+\frac{a+b}{2}+\frac{c+b}{2}=a+b+c$$

That is, $\frac{a^2}{b+c}+\frac{b^2}{c+a}+\frac{c^2}{a+b}\geq\frac{a+b+c}{2}$ or $\frac{2a^2}{b+c}+\frac{2b^2}{c+a}+\frac{2c^2}{a+b}\geq a+b+c$.

Example 7. Let *a, b, c,* be nonnegative real numbers. Show that $\frac{a^3}{b+c}+\frac{b^3}{c+a}+\frac{c^3}{a+b}\geq\frac{a^2+b^2+c^2}{2}$.

Solution:

Method 1:

Since the expression is a symmetric function of a, b and c, we can assume, without loss of generality, that $a\leq b\leq c$. $a^3\leq b^3\leq c^3$. We also see that

$$\frac{1}{b+c}\leq\frac{1}{c+a}\leq\frac{1}{a+b}$$

Then we have the following two similarly ordered sequences:

$a^3,\ b^3,\ c^3,$.

$\frac{1}{b+c},\frac{1}{c+a},\frac{1}{a+b}$

By the rearrangement inequality, we have

$$\begin{array}{ccccccc} a^3 & b^3 & c^3 & a^3 & b^3 & c^3 & a^3 \\ \downarrow & \downarrow & \downarrow & \nearrow & \nearrow & \nearrow & \\ \frac{1}{b+c} & \frac{1}{c+a} & \frac{1}{a+b} & \frac{1}{b+c} & \frac{1}{c+a} & \frac{1}{a+b} & \frac{1}{b+c} \end{array}$$

$$\frac{a^3}{b+c}+\frac{b^3}{c+a}+\frac{c^3}{a+b}\geq \frac{b^3}{b+c}+\frac{c^3}{c+a}+\frac{a^3}{a+b} \qquad (1)$$

$$\begin{array}{ccccccc} a^3 & b^3 & c^3 & a^3 & b^3 & c^3 & a^3 \\ \downarrow & \downarrow & \downarrow & \searrow & \searrow & \searrow & \\ \frac{1}{b+c} & \frac{1}{c+a} & \frac{1}{a+b} & \frac{1}{b+c} & \frac{1}{c+a} & \frac{1}{a+b} & \frac{1}{b+c} \end{array}$$

$$\frac{a^3}{b+c}+\frac{b^3}{c+a}+\frac{c^3}{a+b}\geq \frac{c^3}{b+c}+\frac{a^3}{c+a}+\frac{b^3}{a+b} \qquad (2)$$

(1) + (2):

$$2\left(\frac{a^3}{b+c}+\frac{b^3}{c+a}+\frac{c^3}{a+b}\right)\geq \frac{c^3+b^3}{b+c}+\frac{a^3+c^3}{c+a}+\frac{b^3+a^3}{a+b}$$

$$= c^2-cb+b^2+a^2-ac+c^2+b^2-ba+a^2$$

$$= 2(a^2+b^2+c^2)-(ca+ab+ba) \qquad (3)$$

We know from AM-GM that $ca+ab+ba\leq a^2+b^2+c^2$

(3) can be written as:

$$2\left(\frac{a^3}{b+c}+\frac{b^3}{c+a}+\frac{c^3}{a+b}\right)\geq 2(a^2+b^2+c^2)-(a^2+b^2+c^2)$$

or $\frac{a^3}{b+c}+\frac{b^3}{c+a}+\frac{c^3}{a+b}\geq\frac{a^2+b^2+c^2}{2}$.

Method 2:

The left-hand side of the given inequality can be written as

$$\frac{a^3}{b+c}+\frac{b^3}{c+a}+\frac{c^3}{a+b}=\frac{a^4}{a(b+c)}+\frac{b^4}{b(c+a)}+\frac{c^4}{c(a+b)}.$$

By Cauchy, we have

$$\frac{a^4}{a(b+c)}+\frac{b^4}{b(c+a)}+\frac{c^4}{c(a+b)}\geq\frac{(a^2+b^2+b^2)^2}{2(ab+bc+ca)} \qquad (1)$$

We know from AM-GM that $ca+ab+ba\leq a^2+b^2+c^2$

(1) can be written as

$$\frac{a^4}{a(b+c)}+\frac{b^4}{b(c+a)}+\frac{c^4}{c(a+b)}\geq\frac{(a^2+b^2+b^2)^2}{2(a^2+b^2+c^2)}=\frac{a^2+b^2+c^2}{2}.$$

Example 8. (2005 Romania) Let *a, b, c* be positive real numbers. Prove that

$$\frac{b+c}{a^2}+\frac{c+a}{b^2}+\frac{a+b}{c^2}\geq\frac{1}{a}+\frac{1}{b}+\frac{1}{c}.$$

Proof:

Method 1:

Since the inequality is symmetric, WLOG, we may assume that $a\leq b\leq c$.

For the following similarly sorted sequences,

a, b, c

$\frac{1}{c^2}, \frac{1}{b^2}, \frac{1}{a^2}$

by the rearrangement inequality, we have

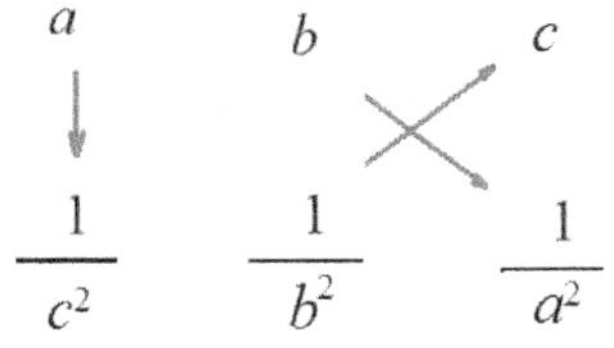

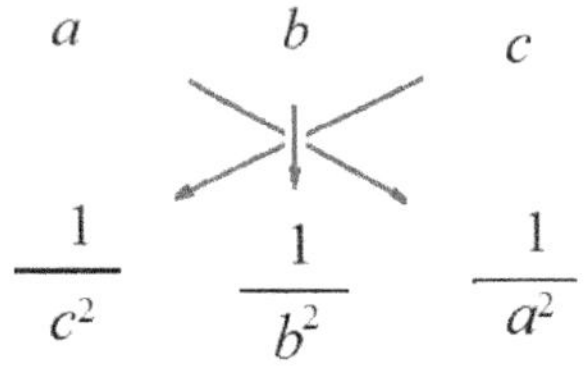

$$a \quad b \quad c \qquad\qquad a \quad b \quad c$$

$$\frac{1}{c^2} \quad \frac{1}{b^2} \quad \frac{1}{a^2} \qquad\qquad \frac{1}{c^2} \quad \frac{1}{b^2} \quad \frac{1}{a^2}$$

$$\frac{a}{c^2}+\frac{b}{a^2}+\frac{c}{b^2}\geq\frac{a}{a^2}+\frac{b}{b^2}+\frac{c}{c^2}=\frac{1}{a}+\frac{1}{b}+\frac{1}{c} \qquad (2)$$

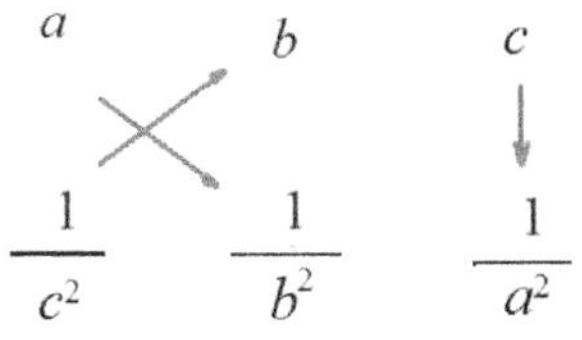

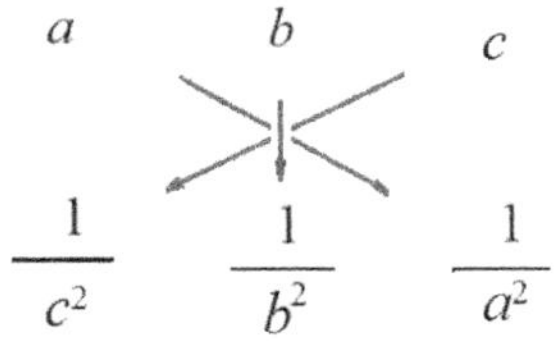

$$a \quad b \quad c \qquad\qquad a \quad b \quad c$$

$$\frac{1}{c^2} \quad \frac{1}{b^2} \quad \frac{1}{a^2} \qquad\qquad \frac{1}{c^2} \quad \frac{1}{b^2} \quad \frac{1}{a^2}$$

$$\frac{a}{b^2}+\frac{b}{c^2}+\frac{c}{a^2}\geq\frac{a}{a^2}+\frac{b}{b^2}+\frac{c}{c^2}=\frac{1}{a}+\frac{1}{b}+\frac{1}{c} \qquad (2)$$

(1) + (2):
$\frac{a}{c^2}+\frac{b}{a^2}+\frac{c}{b^2}+\frac{a}{b^2}+\frac{b}{c^2}+\frac{c}{a^2}=\frac{b+c}{a^2}+\frac{c+a}{b^2}+\frac{a+b}{c^2}\geq 2(\frac{1}{a}+\frac{1}{b}+\frac{1}{c})\geq \frac{1}{a}+\frac{1}{b}+\frac{1}{c}$.

Method 2:

By using the Cauchy inequality we have

$$(\frac{1}{a}+\frac{1}{b}+\frac{1}{c})^2=(\frac{\sqrt{b+c}}{a}\cdot\frac{1}{\sqrt{b+c}}+\frac{\sqrt{c+a}}{b}\cdot\frac{1}{\sqrt{c+a}}+\frac{\sqrt{a+b}}{c}\cdot\frac{1}{\sqrt{a+b}})^2$$

$$\leq\left(\frac{b+c}{a^2}+\frac{c+a}{b^2}+\frac{a+b}{c^2}\right)(\frac{1}{b+c}+\frac{1}{c+a}+\frac{1}{a+b})$$

$$\leq\left(\frac{b+c}{a^2}+\frac{c+a}{b^2}+\frac{a+b}{c^2}\right)(\frac{1}{a}+\frac{1}{b}+\frac{1}{c}).$$

Thus, $\frac{b+c}{a^2}+\frac{c+a}{b^2}+\frac{a+b}{c^2}\geq\frac{1}{a}+\frac{1}{b}+\frac{1}{c}$.

Example 9. (2005 Serbia Math Olympiad) For positive numbers a, b, c, prove that $\frac{a}{\sqrt{b+c}}+\frac{b}{\sqrt{c+a}}+\frac{c}{\sqrt{a+b}}\geq\sqrt{\frac{3}{2}(a+b+c)}$.

Solution:

Method 1:

$$\frac{a}{\sqrt{b+c}}+\frac{b}{\sqrt{c+a}}+\frac{c}{\sqrt{a+b}}=\frac{a^2}{a\sqrt{b+c}}+\frac{b^2}{b\sqrt{c+a}}+\frac{c^2}{c\sqrt{a+b}}$$

$$\geq\frac{(a+b+c)^2}{a\sqrt{b+c}+b\sqrt{a+c}+c\sqrt{a+b}}\qquad(1)$$

Since the inequality is symmetric, WLOG, we may assume that $a\leq b\leq c$. Then we know that $\sqrt{a+b}\leq\sqrt{a+c}\leq\sqrt{b+c}$

Then we have the following two similarly ordered sequences:

$a\,,b\,,c$

$\sqrt{a+b}\,,\sqrt{a+c}\,,\sqrt{b+c}$

By the rearrangement inequality, we have

$a \quad b \quad c \qquad\qquad a \quad b \quad c$

$\sqrt{a+b} \;\; \sqrt{a+c} \;\; \sqrt{b+c} \qquad \sqrt{a+b} \;\; \sqrt{a+c} \;\; \sqrt{b+c}$

$$a\sqrt{b+c} + b\sqrt{a+c} + c\sqrt{a+b} \le c\sqrt{a+b} + b\sqrt{a+c} + a\sqrt{b+c} \qquad (2)$$

$a \quad b \quad c \qquad\qquad a \quad b \quad c$

$\sqrt{a+b} \;\; \sqrt{a+c} \;\; \sqrt{b+c} \qquad \sqrt{a+b} \;\; \sqrt{a+c} \;\; \sqrt{b+c}$

$$a\sqrt{b+c} + b\sqrt{a+c} + c\sqrt{a+b} \le b\sqrt{a+b} + a\sqrt{a+c} + c\sqrt{b+c} \qquad (3)$$

We also have

$$a\sqrt{b+c} + b\sqrt{a+c} + c\sqrt{a+b} \le a\sqrt{b+c} + b\sqrt{a+c} + c\sqrt{a+b} \qquad (4)$$

(2) + (3) + (4):

$$3(a\sqrt{b+c} + b\sqrt{a+c} + c\sqrt{a+b}) \le (a+b+c)(\sqrt{a+b} + \sqrt{a+c} + \sqrt{b+c})$$

Or

$$a\sqrt{b+c} + b\sqrt{a+c} + c\sqrt{a+b} \le \frac{1}{3}(a+b+c)(\sqrt{a+b} + \sqrt{a+c} + \sqrt{b+c})$$

$$\le \frac{1}{3}(a+b+c)(\sqrt{3[(a+b)+a+c)+(b+c)]}$$

$$= \frac{\sqrt{6}}{3}(a+b+c)^{\frac{3}{2}} \qquad (5)$$

Substituting (5) into (1):

$$\frac{a^2}{a\sqrt{b+c}} + \frac{b^2}{b\sqrt{c+a}} + \frac{c^2}{c\sqrt{a+b}} \ge \frac{(a+b+c)^2}{\frac{\sqrt{6}}{3}(a+b+c)^{\frac{3}{2}}} = \sqrt{\frac{3}{2}(a+b+c)}$$. QED.

Method 2:

Since the inequality is homogenous, we may assume, WLOG, that $abc = 1$. Thus by AM-GM, $a + b + c \ge 3\sqrt[3]{abc} = 3$.

The given inequality becomes: $\frac{a}{\sqrt{b+c}}+\frac{b}{\sqrt{c+a}}+\frac{c}{\sqrt{a+b}}\ge\frac{3\sqrt{2}}{2}$.

We have the following two similarly ordered sequences:
a, b, c.
$\frac{1}{\sqrt{b+c}}, \frac{1}{\sqrt{c+a}}, \frac{1}{\sqrt{a+b}}$

By the rearrangement inequality, we have

$$\begin{array}{ccc} a & b & c \\ \downarrow & \downarrow & \downarrow \\ \frac{1}{\sqrt{b+c}} & \frac{1}{\sqrt{a+c}} & \frac{1}{\sqrt{a+b}} \end{array} \qquad \begin{array}{cccc} a & b & c & a \\ \searrow & \searrow & \searrow & \\ \frac{1}{\sqrt{b+c}} & \frac{1}{\sqrt{a+c}} & \frac{1}{\sqrt{a+b}} & \frac{1}{\sqrt{b+c}} \end{array}$$

$$\frac{a}{\sqrt{b+c}}+\frac{b}{\sqrt{c+a}}+\frac{c}{\sqrt{a+b}}\ge\frac{a}{\sqrt{a+c}}+\frac{b}{\sqrt{a+b}}+\frac{c}{\sqrt{b+c}} \qquad (1)$$

$$\begin{array}{ccc} a & b & c \\ \downarrow & \downarrow & \downarrow \\ \frac{1}{\sqrt{b+c}} & \frac{1}{\sqrt{a+c}} & \frac{1}{\sqrt{a+b}} \end{array} \qquad \begin{array}{cccc} a & b & c & a \\ \nearrow & \nearrow & \nearrow & \\ \frac{1}{\sqrt{b+c}} & \frac{1}{\sqrt{a+c}} & \frac{1}{\sqrt{a+b}} & \frac{1}{\sqrt{b+c}} \end{array}$$

$$\frac{a}{\sqrt{b+c}}+\frac{b}{\sqrt{c+a}}+\frac{c}{\sqrt{a+b}}\ge\frac{b}{\sqrt{b+c}}+\frac{c}{\sqrt{c+a}}+\frac{a}{\sqrt{a+b}} \qquad (2)$$

(1) + (2):

$$2\left(\frac{a}{\sqrt{b+c}}+\frac{b}{\sqrt{c+a}}+\frac{c}{\sqrt{a+b}}\right)\ge\frac{a+c}{\sqrt{a+c}}+\frac{b+a}{\sqrt{a+b}}+\frac{c+b}{\sqrt{b+c}}$$
$$=\sqrt{a+c}+\sqrt{b+a}+\sqrt{c+b}$$

We see that $\sqrt{a+b}+\sqrt{a+c}+\sqrt{b+c}$

$$\ge 3\sqrt[3]{\sqrt{(a+b)(b+c)(c+a)}}\ge 3\sqrt[3]{\sqrt{8abc}}=3\sqrt[3]{\sqrt{2^3}}=3\sqrt[6]{2^3}=3\sqrt{2}.$$

We have $2\left(\frac{a}{\sqrt{b+c}}+\frac{b}{\sqrt{c+a}}+\frac{c}{\sqrt{a+b}}\right)\ge 3\sqrt{2}$ or

$\frac{a}{\sqrt{b+c}}+\frac{b}{\sqrt{c+a}}+\frac{c}{\sqrt{a+b}}\geq\frac{3\sqrt{2}}{2}$ QED.

Example 10. (31st IMO Shortlisted) Let a, b, c, d be nonnegative real numbers such that $ab+bc+cd+da=1$. Show that $\frac{a^3}{b+c+d}+\frac{b^3}{c+d+a}+\frac{c^3}{d+a+b}+\frac{d^3}{a+b+c}\geq\frac{1}{3}$.

Solution:

Method 1:

Since the expression is a symmetric function of a, b and c, we can assume, without loss of generality, that $a\leq b\leq c\leq d$. $a^3\leq b^3\leq c^3\leq d^3$. We also see that

$$\frac{1}{b+c+d}\leq\frac{1}{c+d+a}\leq\frac{1}{d+a+b}\leq\frac{1}{a+b+c}$$

Then we have the following two similarly ordered sequences:

$a^3,\ b^3,\ c^3,\ d^3.$

$\frac{1}{b+c+d},\frac{1}{c+d+a},\frac{1}{d+a+b},\frac{1}{a+b+c}$

By the rearrangement inequality, we have

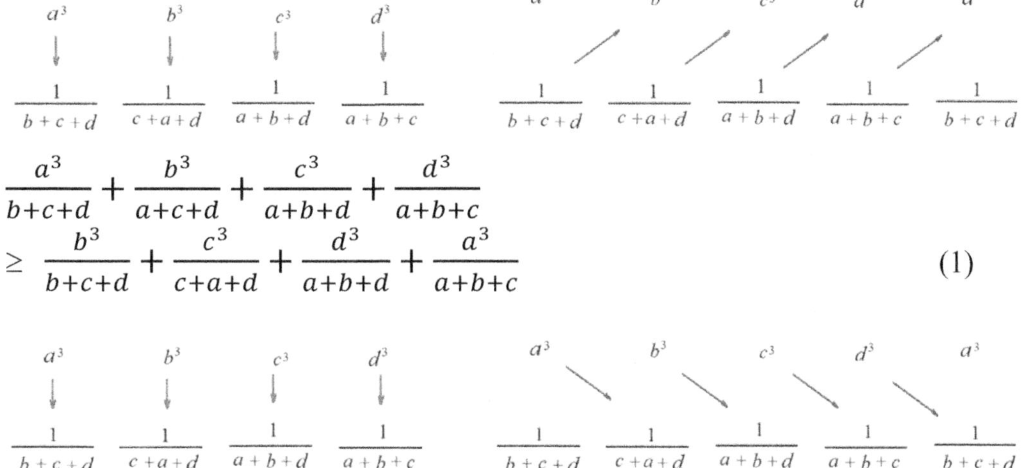

$$\frac{a^3}{b+c+d}+\frac{b^3}{a+c+d}+\frac{c^3}{a+b+d}+\frac{d^3}{a+b+c}$$

$$\geq\frac{b^3}{b+c+d}+\frac{c^3}{c+a+d}+\frac{d^3}{a+b+d}+\frac{a^3}{a+b+c} \qquad (1)$$

$$\frac{a^3}{b+c+d}+\frac{b^3}{a+c+d}+\frac{c^3}{a+b+d}+\frac{d^3}{a+b+c}$$
$$\geq \frac{d^3}{b+c+d}+\frac{a^3}{c+a+d}+\frac{b^3}{a+b+d}+\frac{c^3}{a+b+c} \qquad (2)$$

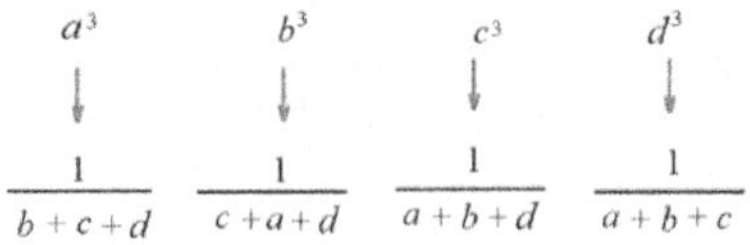

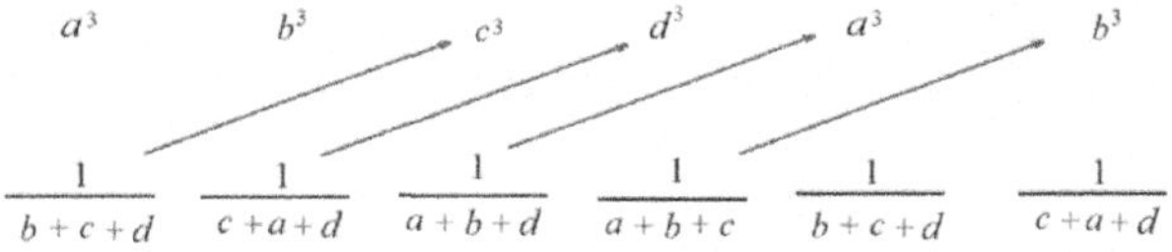

$$\begin{array}{cccc} a^3 & b^3 & c^3 & d^3 \\ \downarrow & \downarrow & \downarrow & \downarrow \\ \frac{1}{b+c+d} & \frac{1}{c+a+d} & \frac{1}{a+b+d} & \frac{1}{a+b+c} \end{array} \qquad \begin{array}{cccccc} a^3 & b^3 & c^3 & d^3 & a^3 & b^3 \\ \frac{1}{b+c+d} & \frac{1}{c+a+d} & \frac{1}{a+b+d} & \frac{1}{a+b+c} & \frac{1}{b+c+d} & \frac{1}{c+a+d} \end{array}$$

$$\frac{a^3}{b+c+d}+\frac{b^3}{a+c+d}+\frac{c^3}{a+b+d}+\frac{d^3}{a+b+c}$$
$$\geq \frac{c^3}{b+c+d}+\frac{d^3}{c+a+d}+\frac{a^3}{a+b+d}+\frac{b^3}{a+b+c} \qquad (3)$$

(1) + (2) + (3):

$$3(\frac{a^3}{b+c+d}+\frac{b^3}{a+c+d}+\frac{c^3}{a+b+d}+\frac{d^3}{a+b+c})$$
$$\geq \frac{a^3+b^3+c^3}{a+b+c}+\frac{b^3+c^3+d^3}{b+c+d}+\frac{c^3+d^3+a^3}{c+d+a}+\frac{d^3+a^3+b^3}{d+a+b} \qquad (4)$$

We know from AM-GM that $3(a^3+b^3+c^3)\geq(a+b+c)(a^2+b^2+c^2)$.

(4) can be written as:

$$3(\frac{a^3}{b+c+d}+\frac{b^3}{c+d+a}+\frac{c^3}{d+a+b}+\frac{d^3}{a+b+c})\geq a^2+b^2+c^2+d^2 \qquad (5)$$

Also by the AM-GM inequality $a^2+b^2+c^2+d^2\geq ab+bc+cd+da=1$, we have $\frac{a^3}{b+c+d}+\frac{b^3}{c+d+a}+\frac{c^3}{d+a+b}+\frac{d^3}{a+b+c}\geq\frac{1}{3}$.

Method 2:

Since the expression is a symmetric function of a, b and c, we can assume, without loss of generality, that $a\leq b\leq c\leq d$. We also see that

$$\frac{a^2}{b+c+d}\leq\frac{b^2}{c+d+a}\leq\frac{c^2}{d+a+b}\leq\frac{d^2}{a+b+c}$$

Then we have the following two similarly ordered sequences:

$a,\ b,\ c,\ d$.

$$\frac{a^2}{b+c+d}, \frac{b^2}{c+d+a}, \frac{c^2}{d+a+b}, \frac{d^2}{a+b+c}$$

By the rearrangement inequality

a ↓ $\frac{a^2}{b+c+d}$ b ↓ $\frac{b^2}{c+d+a}$ c ↓ $\frac{c^2}{d+a+b}$ d ↓ $\frac{d^2}{a+b+c}$ a $\frac{a^2}{b+c+d}$ b $\frac{b^2}{c+d+a}$ c $\frac{c^2}{d+a+b}$ d $\frac{d^2}{a+b+c}$ a $\frac{a^2}{b+c+d}$

a ↓ $\frac{a^2}{b+c+d}$ b ↓ $\frac{b^2}{c+d+a}$ c ↓ $\frac{c^2}{d+a+b}$ d ↓ $\frac{d^2}{a+b+c}$ a $\frac{a^2}{b+c+d}$ b $\frac{b^2}{c+d+a}$ c $\frac{c^2}{d+a+b}$ d $\frac{d^2}{a+b+c}$ a $\frac{a^2}{b+c+d}$

a ↓ $\frac{a^2}{b+c+d}$ b ↓ $\frac{b^2}{c+d+a}$ c ↓ $\frac{c^2}{d+a+b}$ d ↓ $\frac{d^2}{a+b+c}$ a b c d $\frac{a^2}{b+c+d}$ $\frac{b^2}{c+d+a}$ $\frac{c^2}{d+a+b}$ $\frac{d^2}{a+b+c}$

$$\frac{a^3}{b+c+d}+\frac{b^3}{c+d+a}+\frac{c^3}{d+a+b}+\frac{d^3}{a+b+c}$$
$$\geq \frac{ab^2}{c+d+a}+\frac{bc^2}{d+a+b}+\frac{cd^2}{a+b+c}+\frac{da^2}{b+c+d} \qquad (1)$$

$$\frac{a^3}{b+c+d}+\frac{b^3}{c+d+a}+\frac{c^3}{d+a+b}+\frac{d^3}{a+b+c}$$
$$\geq \frac{ad^2}{a+b+c}+\frac{ba^2}{b+c+d}+\frac{cb^2}{c+d+a}+\frac{dc^2}{d+a+b} \qquad (2)$$

$$\frac{a^3}{b+c+d}+\frac{b^3}{c+d+a}+\frac{c^3}{d+a+b}+\frac{d^3}{a+b+c}$$
$$\geq \frac{ac^2}{d+a+b}+\frac{bd^2}{a+b+c}+\frac{ca^2}{b+c+d}+\frac{db^2}{c+d+a} \qquad (3)$$

(1) + (2) + (3):

$$3\left(\frac{a^3}{b+c+d}+\frac{b^3}{c+d+a}+\frac{c^3}{d+a+b}+\frac{d^3}{a+b+c}\right)$$
$$\geq \frac{da^2+ba^2+ca^2}{b+c+d}+\frac{db^2+cb^2+ab^2}{c+d+a}+\frac{ac^2+bc^2+dc^2}{d+a+b}+\frac{ad^2+bd^2+cd^2}{a+b+c}$$
$$= a^2+b^2+c^2+d^2 \geq ab+bc+cd+da = 1 \qquad (4)$$

Thus $\frac{a^3}{b+c+d}+\frac{b^3}{c+d+a}+\frac{c^3}{d+a+b}+\frac{d^3}{a+b+c}\geq\frac{1}{3}$.

Example 11. (39th IMO Shortlisted) *a, b, c* are positive reals with product 1. Show that $\frac{a^3}{(1+b)(1+c)}+\frac{b^3}{(1+c)(1+a)}+\frac{c^3}{(1+a)(1+b)}\geq\frac{3}{4}$.

Solution:

Since the expression is a symmetric function of *a*, *b* and *c*, we can assume, without loss of generality, that $a\leq b\leq c$. $abc=1$. $a^3\leq b^3\leq c^3$.

$$\frac{1}{(1+b)(1+c)}\leq\frac{1}{(1+c)(1+a)}\leq\frac{1}{(1+a)(1+b)}$$

Then we have the following two similarly ordered sequences:

a^3, b^3, c^3

$$\frac{1}{(1+b)(1+c)},\frac{1}{(1+c)(1+a)},\frac{1}{(1+a)(1+b)}$$

By the rearrangement inequality,

$$\begin{array}{ccc} a^3 & b^3 & c^3 \\ \downarrow & \downarrow & \downarrow \\ \frac{1}{(1+b)(1+c)} & \frac{1}{(1+c)(1+a)} & \frac{1}{(1+a)(1+b)} \end{array} \qquad \begin{array}{cccc} a^3 & b^3 & c^3 & a^3 \\ \searrow & \searrow & \searrow & \\ \frac{1}{(1+b)(1+c)} & \frac{1}{(1+c)(1+a)} & \frac{1}{(1+a)(1+b)} & \frac{1}{(1+b)(1+c)} \end{array}$$

$$\frac{a^3}{(1+b)(1+c)}+\frac{b^3}{(1+c)(1+a)}+\frac{c^3}{(1+a)(1+b)}\geq\frac{a^3}{(1+c)(1+a)}+\frac{b^3}{(1+a)(1+b)}+\frac{c^3}{(1+b)(1+c)} \qquad (1)$$

$$\begin{array}{ccc} a^3 & b^3 & c^3 \\ \downarrow & \downarrow & \downarrow \\ \frac{1}{(1+b)(1+c)} & \frac{1}{(1+c)(1+a)} & \frac{1}{(1+a)(1+b)} \end{array} \qquad \begin{array}{cccc} a^3 & b^3 & c^3 & a^3 \\ \nearrow & \nearrow & \nearrow & \\ \frac{1}{(1+b)(1+c)} & \frac{1}{(1+c)(1+a)} & \frac{1}{(1+a)(1+b)} & \frac{1}{(1+b)(1+c)} \end{array}$$

$$\frac{a^3}{(1+b)(1+c)}+\frac{b^3}{(1+c)(1+a)}+\frac{c^3}{(1+a)(1+b)} \geq \frac{a^3}{(1+a)(1+b)}+\frac{b^3}{(1+b)(1+c)}+\frac{c^3}{(1+c)(1+a)} \qquad (2)$$

a^3	b^3	c^3	a^3	b^3	c^3
$\downarrow$	$\downarrow$	$\downarrow$	$\downarrow$	$\downarrow$	$\downarrow$
$\frac{1}{(1+b)(1+c)}$	$\frac{1}{(1+c)(1+a)}$	$\frac{1}{(1+a)(1+b)}$	$\frac{1}{(1+b)(1+c)}$	$\frac{1}{(1+c)(1+a)}$	$\frac{1}{(1+a)(1+b)}$

$$\frac{a^3}{(1+b)(1+c)}+\frac{b^3}{(1+c)(1+a)}+\frac{c^3}{(1+a)(1+b)} \geq \frac{a^3}{(1+b)(1+c)}+\frac{b^3}{(1+c)(1+a)}+\frac{c^3}{(1+a)(1+b)} \qquad (3)$$

(1) + (2) + (3):

$$3\left(\frac{a^3}{(1+b)(1+c)}+\frac{b^3}{(1+c)(1+a)}+\frac{c^3}{(1+a)(1+b)}\right) \geq \frac{a^3+b^3+c^3}{(1+b)(1+c)}+\frac{a^3+b^3+c^3}{(1+c)(1+a)}+\frac{a^3+b^3+c^3}{(1+a)(1+b)}$$

$$= (a^3+b^3+c^3)\left[\frac{1}{(1+b)(1+c)}+\frac{1}{(1+c)(1+a)}+\frac{1}{(1+a)(1+b)}\right]$$

$$= (a^3+b^3+c^3)\left[\frac{3+a+b+c}{(1+a)(1+b)(1+c)}\right]$$

Let $m = \frac{1}{3}(a+b+c)$

$$\frac{1}{(1+a)(1+b)(1+c)} \leq \left(\frac{3+a+b+c}{3}\right)^3 = (1+m)^3$$

$a^3+b^3+c^3 \geq 3m^3$.

$a+b+c \geq 3$

$$\frac{a^3}{(1+b)(1+c)}+\frac{b^3}{(1+c)(1+a)}+\frac{c^3}{(1+a)(1+b)}$$

$$\geq \frac{1}{3}(a^3+b^3+c^3)\left[\frac{3+a+b+c}{(1+a)(1+b)(1+c)}\right] = m^3 \cdot \frac{6}{(1+m)^3}.$$

So we only need to prove $m^3 \cdot \frac{6}{(1+m)^3} \geq \frac{3}{4}$.

Since $m \geq 1$, $m^3 \cdot \frac{6}{(1+m)^3} = 6\left(1-\frac{1}{1+m}\right)^3 \geq \frac{3}{4}$.

Equality holds when $a = b = c = 1$.

CHAPTER 6. PROBLEMS

Problem 1. For nonnegative numbers a, b, c, with $abc = 1$, show that $a^2 + b^2 + c^2 \geq a + b + c$.

Problem 2. Let a, b, and c be non-negative real numbers satisfying $a \leq b \leq c$ and $a + b + c = 3$. Show that $ab^2 + bc^2 + ca^2 \leq 4$.

Problem 3. If $a, b, c, d \geq 0$, show that $a^4 + b^4 + c^4 + d^4 \geq 4abcd$.

Problem 4. Prove that for all positive real numbers a, b, c, $\frac{b+c}{a} + \frac{c+a}{b} + \frac{a+b}{c} \geq 6$.

Problem 5. Let $a, b, c > 0$ be real numbers such that $ab + bc + ca = 1$. Prove the Inequality $\frac{a^2}{b+c} + \frac{b^2}{c+a} + \frac{c^2}{a+b} \geq \frac{\sqrt{3}}{2}$.

Problem 6. Let $a, b, c > 0$ be real numbers. Prove the inequality $\frac{a}{(b+c)^2} + \frac{b}{(c+a)^2} + \frac{c}{(a+b)^2} \geq \frac{9}{4(a+b+c)}$.

Problem 7. Let $0 \leq a, b, c \leq 1$. Prove the inequality $\frac{a}{bc+1} + \frac{b}{ca+1} + \frac{c}{ab+1} \leq 2$.

Problem 8. Let a, b, c be nonnegative real numbers. Show that $\frac{a^3}{b+c} + \frac{b^3}{c+a} + \frac{c^3}{a+b} \geq \frac{ca+ab+ba}{2}$.

Problem 9. (2005 Romania, unused) For positive numbers a, b, c, $a + b + c = 1$, prove that $\frac{a}{\sqrt{b+c}} + \frac{b}{\sqrt{c+a}} + \frac{c}{\sqrt{a+b}} \ge \sqrt{\frac{3}{2}}$.

Problem 10. (2018 French JBMO) If $0 \le a \le b \le c \le d$, show that $ab^3 + bc^3 + cd^3 + da^3 \ge a^2b^2 + b^2c^2 + c^2d^2 + d^2a^2$.

Problem 11. Let a, b, c be positive real numbers such that $abc = 1$. Show that

$$\frac{a^3}{2a^3+b^3+c^3} + \frac{b^3}{2b^3+c^3+a^3} + \frac{c^3}{2c^3+a^3+b^3} \le \frac{\sqrt{a}+\sqrt{b}+\sqrt{c}}{4}.$$

Problem 12. a and b are positive integers such that $a + b \le 2ab$. Prove that $\frac{a}{a^2+b} + \frac{b}{b^2+a} \le 1$.

CHAPTER 6. SOLUTIONS

Problem 1. Proof:

Method 1:

For the following similarly ordered sequences,

$a, \ b, c$

a, b, c

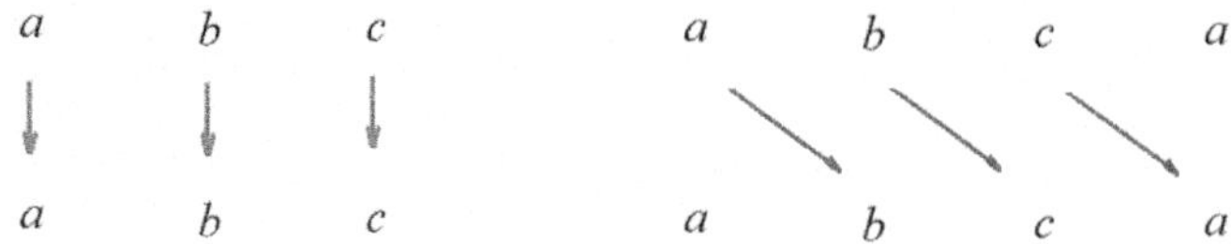

By the rearrangement inequality, we have

$a^2 + b^2 + c^2 \geq ab + bc + ca$ (1)

(1) × 2: $2(a^2 + b^2 + c^2) \geq 2(ab + bc + ca)$ (2)

Adding $a^2 + b^2 + c^2$ to both sides of (2):

$3(a^2 + b^2 + c^2) \geq a^2 + b^2 + c^2 + 2ab + 2bc + 2ca = (a + b + c)^2$

$= \ (a + b + c)(a + b + c)$

$\geq 3\sqrt[3]{abc}\,(a + b + c) = 3(a + b + c)$.

Thus $a^2 + b^2 + c^2 \geq a + b + c$. QED.

Method 2:

Since $abc = 1$, we have $\sqrt[3]{abc} = \sqrt[3]{a} \cdot \sqrt[3]{b} \cdot \sqrt[3]{c} = 1$.

We have the following similarly ordered sequences,

$\sqrt[3]{a}, \sqrt[3]{b}, \sqrt[3]{c}$

$\sqrt[3]{a}, \sqrt[3]{b}, \sqrt[3]{c}$

$\sqrt[3]{a^4}, \sqrt[3]{b^4}, \sqrt[3]{c^4},$

By the rearrangement inequality, we have

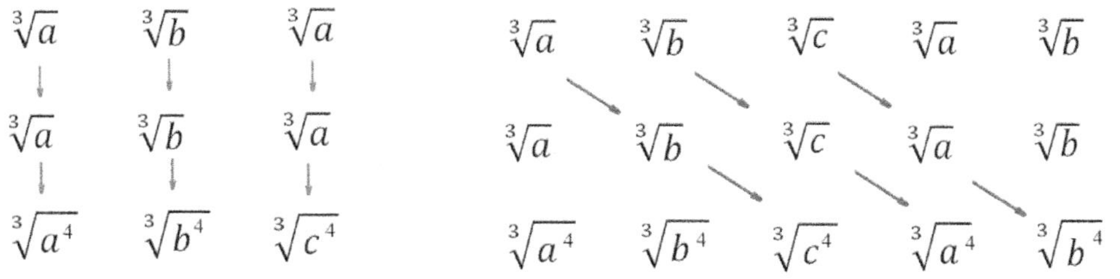

$$\begin{matrix} \sqrt[3]{a} & \sqrt[3]{b} & \sqrt[3]{a} \\ \downarrow & \downarrow & \downarrow \\ \sqrt[3]{a} & \sqrt[3]{b} & \sqrt[3]{a} \\ \downarrow & \downarrow & \downarrow \\ \sqrt[3]{a^4} & \sqrt[3]{b^4} & \sqrt[3]{c^4} \end{matrix} \qquad \begin{matrix} \sqrt[3]{a} & \sqrt[3]{b} & \sqrt[3]{c} & \sqrt[3]{a} & \sqrt[3]{b} \\ \sqrt[3]{a} & \sqrt[3]{b} & \sqrt[3]{c} & \sqrt[3]{a} & \sqrt[3]{b} \\ \sqrt[3]{a^4} & \sqrt[3]{b^4} & \sqrt[3]{c^4} & \sqrt[3]{a^4} & \sqrt[3]{b^4} \end{matrix}$$

or $\begin{bmatrix} \sqrt[3]{a} & \sqrt[3]{b} & \sqrt[3]{c} \\ \sqrt[3]{a} & \sqrt[3]{b} & \sqrt[3]{c} \\ \sqrt[3]{a^4} & \sqrt[3]{b^4} & \sqrt[3]{c^4} \end{bmatrix} \geq \begin{bmatrix} \sqrt[3]{a} & \sqrt[3]{b} & \sqrt[3]{c} \\ \sqrt[3]{b} & \sqrt[3]{c} & \sqrt[3]{a} \\ \sqrt[3]{c^4} & \sqrt[3]{a^4} & \sqrt[3]{b^4} \end{bmatrix}$

$\sqrt[3]{a}\cdot\sqrt[3]{a}\cdot\sqrt[3]{a^4}+\sqrt[3]{b}\cdot\sqrt[3]{b}\cdot\sqrt[3]{b^4}+\sqrt[3]{c}\cdot\sqrt[3]{c}\cdot\sqrt[3]{c^4}$
$\geq \sqrt[3]{a}\cdot\sqrt[3]{b}\cdot\sqrt[3]{c^4}+\sqrt[3]{b}\cdot\sqrt[3]{c}\cdot\sqrt[3]{a^4}+\sqrt[3]{c}\cdot\sqrt[3]{a}\cdot\sqrt[3]{b^4} \qquad \Rightarrow$
$\sqrt[3]{a^6}+\sqrt[3]{b^6}+\sqrt[3]{c^6} \geq \sqrt[3]{a}\cdot\sqrt[3]{b}\cdot\sqrt[3]{c}\cdot\sqrt[3]{c^3}+\sqrt[3]{b}\cdot\sqrt[3]{c}\cdot\sqrt[3]{a}\cdot\sqrt[3]{a^3}+\sqrt[3]{c}\cdot\sqrt[3]{a}\cdot\sqrt[3]{b}\cdot$
$\sqrt[3]{b^3}$

Thus $a^2 + b^2 + c^2 \geq a + b + c$. QED.

Note: for any positive integer n, $abc = 1$: $3 \leq a + b + c \leq a^2 + b^2 + c^2 \leq a^3 +$
$b^3 + c^3 \leq a^4 + b^4 + c^4 \leq \ldots \leq a^n + b^n + c^n$.

Problem 2. Solution:
Since $a \leq b \leq c$, we have $ab \leq ac \leq bc$.
Then we have the following two similarly ordered sequences:
a, b, c
ab, ac, bc.

By the rearrangement inequality,

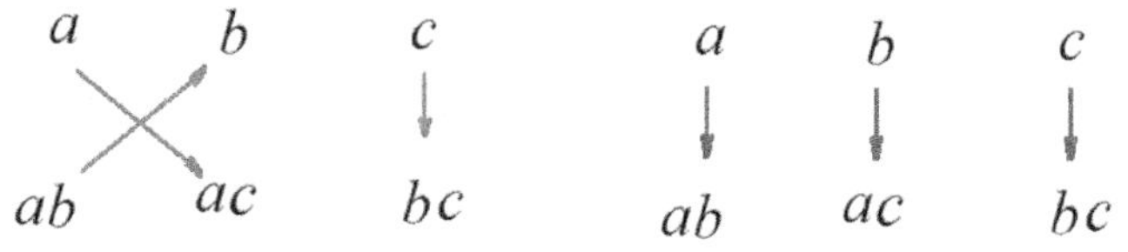

$$\begin{matrix} a & b & c \\ \searrow\!\!\!\!\nearrow & & \downarrow \\ ab & ac & bc \end{matrix} \qquad \begin{matrix} a & b & c \\ \downarrow & \downarrow & \downarrow \\ ab & ac & bc \end{matrix}$$

$ab^2 + bc^2 + ca^2 \leq a^2b + abc + c^2b = b(a^2 + ac + c^2)$

$\leq b(a+c)^2 = \frac{1}{2}(2b)(a+c)(a+c) \leq \frac{1}{2}(\frac{2b+(a+c)+(a+c)}{3})^3 = \frac{1}{2}(\frac{2\cdot 3}{3})^3 = \frac{8}{2} = 4.$

We are done. Equality holds for $a = 1$, $b = 2$, $c = 0$ and its permutations.

Problem 3. Solution:

Method 1:

Since the inequality is symmetric, WLOG, we may assume that

$a \leq b \leq c \leq d.$

For the following two similarly ordered sequences,

a, b, c, d

$a^3, b^3 c^3, d^3$

by the shoelace inequality,

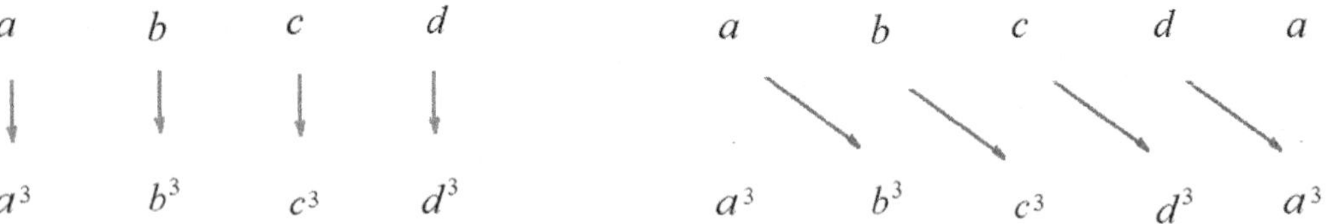

$a^4 + b^4 + c^4 + d^4 \geq ab^3 + bc^3 + cd^3 + da^3 \quad (1)$

Applying AM-GM to the right-hand side of (1):

$$ab^3 + bc^3 + cd^3 + da^3 \geq 4\sqrt[4]{ab^3 \cdot bc^3 \cdot cd^3 \cdot da^3} = 4abcd.$$

Thus $a^4 + b^4 + c^4 + d^4 \geq 4abcd$.

Method 2:

Assume that $a \leq b \leq c \leq d$. Applying the rearrangement to the sequences (c, d) and (c^3, d^3) we obtain

$dc^3 + cd^3 \leq c^4 + d^4.$

Applying the same inequality to the sequences (b, d) and (b^3, cd^2) we obtain $db^3 + bcd^2 \leq b^4 + cd^3$. Together with the previous inequality we have

$db^3 + dc^3 + bcd^2 \leq b^4 + c^4 + d^4.$

We now apply the rearrangement inequality to the sequences (a, d) and (a^3, bcd) to obtain $da^3 + abcd \leq a^4 + bcd^2$ which together with the previous inequality implies

$da^3 + db^3 + dc^3 + abcd \le a^4 + b^4 + c^4 + d^4$.
It suffices to prove $3abcd \le da^3 + db^3 + dc^4$ which is equivalent to $3abc \le a^3 + b^3 + c^3$. For this we use the same argument as before.
Note: See Chapter 2 Problem 6 for another solution.

Problem 4. Solution:
Since the expression is symmetric, WLOG, we can assume that $a \le b \le c$, we know that $a + b \le a + c \le b + c$, $\frac{1}{c} \le \frac{b}{b} \le \frac{1}{a}$.

Then we have the following two similarly ordered sequences:
$a + b, c + a, b + c$,
$\frac{1}{c}, \frac{1}{b}, \frac{1}{a}$.

By the rearrangement inequality, we have

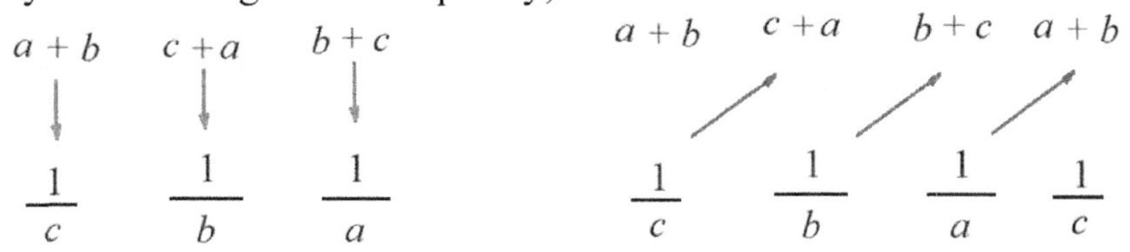

$a+b$	$c+a$	$b+c$
↓	↓	↓
$\frac{1}{c}$	$\frac{1}{b}$	$\frac{1}{a}$

	$a+b$	$c+a$	$b+c$	$a+b$
	↗	↗	↗	
$\frac{1}{c}$	$\frac{1}{b}$	$\frac{1}{a}$	$\frac{1}{c}$	

$$\frac{b+c}{a} + \frac{c+a}{b} + \frac{a+b}{c} \ge \frac{b+a}{a} + \frac{c+b}{b} + \frac{a+c}{c}$$
$$= 3 + \frac{b}{a} + \frac{c}{b} + \frac{a}{c} \ge 3 + 3\sqrt[3]{\frac{b}{a} \cdot \frac{c}{b} \cdot \frac{a}{c}} = 6.$$

Problem 5. Solution:
Since the expression is a symmetric function of a, b and c, we can assume, without loss of generality, that $a \le b \le c$. $a^2 \le b^2 \le c^2$. We also see that
$$\frac{1}{b+c} \le \frac{1}{a+c} \le \frac{1}{a+b}$$

Then we have the following two similarly ordered sequences:
a^2, b^2, c^2
$\frac{1}{b+c}, \frac{1}{c+a}, \frac{1}{a+b}$

By the rearrangement inequality, we have

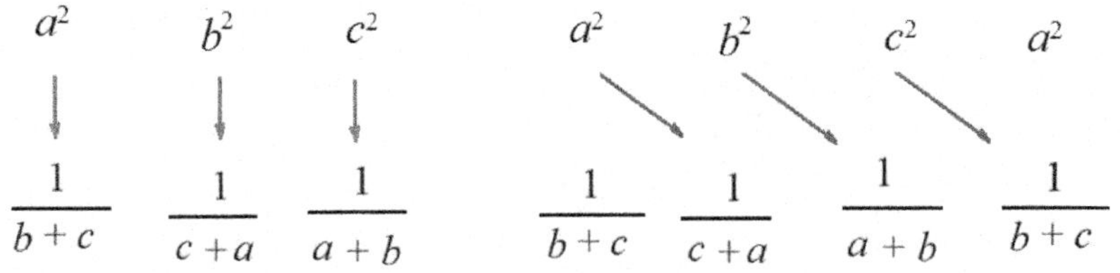

$$\begin{array}{ccc} a^2 & b^2 & c^2 \\ \downarrow & \downarrow & \downarrow \\ \frac{1}{b+c} & \frac{1}{c+a} & \frac{1}{a+b} \end{array} \qquad \begin{array}{cccc} a^2 & b^2 & c^2 & a^2 \\ \searrow & \searrow & \searrow & \\ \frac{1}{b+c} & \frac{1}{c+a} & \frac{1}{a+b} & \frac{1}{b+c} \end{array}$$

$$\frac{a^2}{b+c}+\frac{b^2}{c+a}+\frac{c^2}{a+b}\ge\frac{a^2}{c+a}+\frac{b^2}{a+b}+\frac{c^2}{b+c} \qquad (1)$$

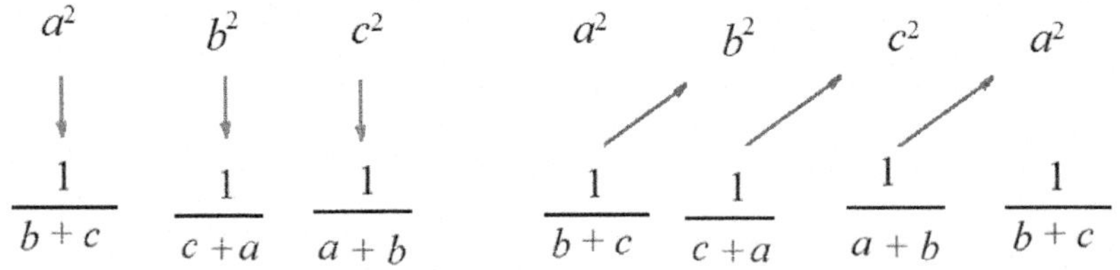

$$\begin{array}{ccc} a^2 & b^2 & c^2 \\ \downarrow & \downarrow & \downarrow \\ \frac{1}{b+c} & \frac{1}{c+a} & \frac{1}{a+b} \end{array} \qquad \begin{array}{cccc} a^2 & b^2 & c^2 & a^2 \\ \nearrow & \nearrow & \nearrow & \\ \frac{1}{b+c} & \frac{1}{c+a} & \frac{1}{a+b} & \frac{1}{b+c} \end{array}$$

$$\frac{a^2}{b+c}+\frac{b^2}{c+a}+\frac{c^2}{a+b}\ge\frac{b^2}{b+c}+\frac{c^2}{c+a}+\frac{a^2}{a+b} \qquad (2)$$

(1) + (2):

$$2\left(\frac{a^2}{b+c}+\frac{b^2}{c+a}+\frac{c^2}{a+b}\right)\ge\frac{a^2+c^2}{c+a}+\frac{b^2+a^2}{a+b}+\frac{c^2+b^2}{b+c}$$

$$\ge\frac{a+c}{2}+\frac{a+b}{2}+\frac{c+b}{2}=a+b+c \qquad (3)$$

Note that

$(a+b+c)^2=a^2+b^2+c^2+2(ab+bc+ca)\ge 3(ab+bc+ca)$
$=3.$

Thus $a+b+c\ge\sqrt{3}$

Substituting this value to (3):

$$2\left(\frac{a^2}{b+c}+\frac{b^2}{c+a}+\frac{c^2}{a+b}\right)\ge a+b+c\ge\sqrt{3}$$

$$\frac{a^2}{b+c}+\frac{b^2}{c+a}+\frac{c^2}{a+b}\ge\frac{\sqrt{3}}{2}.$$

Method 2:

By Cauchy, we have

$$\frac{a^2}{b+c}+\frac{b^2}{c+a}+\frac{c^2}{a+b}\geq\frac{(a+b+c)^2}{2(a+b+c)}=\frac{a+b+c}{2} \qquad (1)$$

Note that
$(a+b+c)^2 = a^2+b^2+c^2+2(ab+bc+ca) \geq 3(ab+bc+ca)$
$= 3.$

Thus $a+b+c \geq \sqrt{3}$

Substituting this value to (1):

$$\frac{a^2}{b+c}+\frac{b^2}{c+a}+\frac{c^2}{a+b}\geq\frac{\sqrt{3}}{2}.$$

Problem 6. Solution:

Since the inequality is symmetrical, WLOG, we can assume that $a \leq b \leq c$, we have the following two similarly ordered sequences:
$a,\ b,\ c$
$\frac{1}{(b+c)^2}, \frac{1}{(c+a)^2}, \frac{1}{(a+b)^2}.$

By the rearrangement inequality, we have

$$\begin{bmatrix} a & b & c \\ \frac{1}{(b+c)^2} & \frac{1}{(c+a)^2} & \frac{1}{(a+b)^2} \end{bmatrix} \geq \begin{bmatrix} a & b & c \\ \frac{1}{(c+a)^2} & \frac{1}{(a+b)^2} & \frac{1}{(b+c)^2} \end{bmatrix}$$

$$\frac{a}{(b+c)^2}+\frac{b}{(c+a)^2}+\frac{c}{(a+b)^2}\geq\frac{a}{(c+a)^2}+\frac{b}{(a+b)^2}+\frac{c}{(b+c)^2} \qquad (1)$$

$$\begin{bmatrix} a & b & c \\ \frac{1}{(b+c)^2} & \frac{1}{(c+a)^2} & \frac{1}{(a+b)^2} \end{bmatrix} \geq \begin{bmatrix} a & b & c \\ \frac{1}{(a+b)^2} & \frac{1}{(b+c)^2} & \frac{1}{(c+a)^2} \end{bmatrix}$$

$$\frac{a}{(b+c)^2}+\frac{b}{(c+a)^2}+\frac{c}{(a+b)^2}\geq\frac{a}{(a+b)^2}+\frac{b}{(b+c)^2}+\frac{c}{(c+a)^2} \qquad (2)$$

(1) + (2):

$$2\left(\frac{a}{(b+c)^2}+\frac{b}{(c+a)^2}+\frac{c}{(a+b)^2}\right)\geq\frac{c+a}{(c+a)^2}+\frac{a+b}{(a+b)^2}+\frac{b+c}{(b+c)^2}=\frac{1}{c+a}+\frac{1}{a+b}+\frac{1}{b+c} \qquad (3)$$

By Cauchy, we have

$$\frac{1}{c+a}+\frac{1}{a+b}+\frac{1}{b+c}\geq\frac{(1+1+1)^2}{2(a+b+c)}=\frac{9}{2(a+b+c)}.$$

Thus $2\left(\frac{a}{(b+c)^2}+\frac{b}{(c+a)^2}+\frac{c}{(a+b)^2}\right)\geq\frac{9}{2(a+b+c)}$ or

$$\frac{a}{(b+c)^2}+\frac{b}{(c+a)^2}+\frac{c}{(a+b)^2}\geq\frac{9}{4(a+b+c)}.$$

Method 2:
Applying Cauchy,

$$(a+b+c)\left(\frac{a}{(b+c)^2}+\frac{b}{(c+a)^2}+\frac{c}{(a+b)^2}\right)\geq\left(\frac{a}{b+c}+\frac{b}{c+a}+\frac{c}{a+b}\right)^2 \qquad (1)$$

Recall Nesbitt's inequality we have

$$\frac{a}{b+c}+\frac{b}{c+a}+\frac{c}{a+b}\geq\frac{3}{2} \qquad (2)$$

Substituting (2) into (1):

$$\frac{a}{(b+c)^2}+\frac{b}{(c+a)^2}+\frac{c}{(a+b)^2}\geq\frac{9}{4(a+b+c)}.$$

Problem 7. Solution:
Since the inequality is symmetrical, WLOG, we can assume that $0\leq a\leq b\leq c\leq 1$, we have the following two similarly ordered sequences:

$a,\ b,\ c$

$\frac{1}{bc+1},\frac{1}{ca+1},\frac{1}{ab+1}.$

By the rearrangement inequality, we see that $\frac{a}{bc+1}+\frac{b}{ca+1}+\frac{c}{ab+1}$ is the largest expression among all possible rearrangements. So we are not able to continue.

$a \quad b \quad c$

$\downarrow \quad \downarrow \quad \downarrow$

$\frac{1}{bc+1} \quad \frac{1}{ac+1} \quad \frac{1}{ab+1}$

However, we see that $0 \le (1-a)(1-b) \le 0$.
Thus we have $a+b \le 1+ab \le 1+2ab \Rightarrow \quad a+b+c \le a+b+1 \le 2(1+ab)$.
Therefore

$$\frac{a}{bc+1}+\frac{b}{ca+1}+\frac{c}{ab+1} \le \frac{a}{ab+1}+\frac{b}{ab+1}+\frac{c}{ab+1} \le \frac{a+b+c}{ab+1} \le \frac{2(1+ab)}{ab+1} = 2.$$

Problem 8. Solution:
Since the expression is a symmetric function of a, b and c, we can assume, without loss of generality, that $a \le b \le c$. $a^3 \le b^3 \le c^3$. We also see that $\frac{1}{b+c} \le \frac{1}{c+a} \le \frac{1}{a+b}$

Then we have the following two similarly ordered sequences:
$a^3,\ b^3,\ c^3,.$
$\frac{1}{b+c}, \frac{1}{c+a}, \frac{1}{a+b}$

By the rearrangement inequality, we have

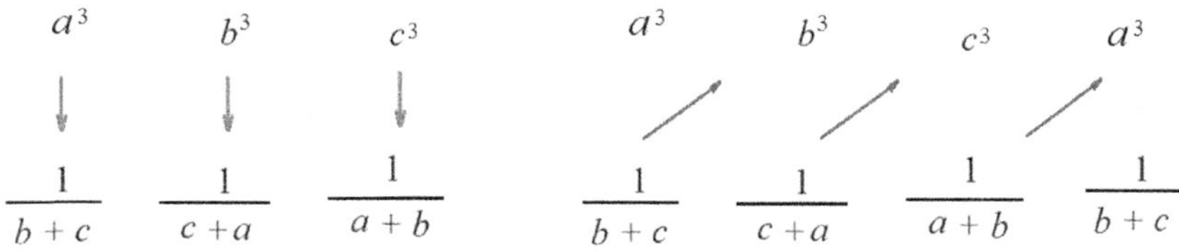

$$\frac{a^3}{b+c}+\frac{b^3}{c+a}+\frac{c^3}{a+b}\geq \frac{b^3}{b+c}+\frac{c^3}{c+a}+\frac{a^3}{a+b} \quad (1)$$

a^3	b^3	c^3		a^3	b^3	c^3	a^3
↓	↓	↓		↘	↘	↘	
$\frac{1}{b+c}$	$\frac{1}{c+a}$	$\frac{1}{a+b}$		$\frac{1}{b+c}$	$\frac{1}{c+a}$	$\frac{1}{a+b}$	$\frac{1}{b+c}$

$$\frac{a^3}{b+c}+\frac{b^3}{c+a}+\frac{c^3}{a+b}\geq \frac{c^3}{b+c}+\frac{a^3}{c+a}+\frac{b^3}{a+b} \quad (2)$$

(1) + (2)):

$$2\left(\frac{a^3}{b+c}+\frac{b^3}{c+a}+\frac{c^3}{a+b}\right)\geq \frac{c^3+b^3}{b+c}+\frac{a^3+c^3}{c+a}+\frac{b^3+a^3}{a+b}$$
$$= c^2-cb+b^2+a^2-ac+c^2+b^2-ba+a^2$$
$$= 2(a^2+b^2+c^2)-(ca+ab+ba) \quad (3)$$

We know from AM-GM that $ca+ab+ba \leq a^2+b^2+c^2$

(3) can be written as:

$$2\left(\frac{a^3}{b+c}+\frac{b^3}{c+a}+\frac{c^3}{a+b}\right)\geq 2(ca+ab+ba)-(ca+ab+ba)$$

or $\frac{a^3}{b+c}+\frac{b^3}{c+a}+\frac{c^3}{a+b}\geq \frac{ca+ab+ba}{2}$.

Problem 9. Solution:

$$\frac{a}{\sqrt{b+c}}+\frac{b}{\sqrt{c+a}}+\frac{c}{\sqrt{a+b}}=\frac{a^2}{a\sqrt{b+c}}+\frac{b^2}{b\sqrt{c+a}}+\frac{c^2}{c\sqrt{a+b}}$$
$$\geq \frac{1}{a\sqrt{b+c}+b\sqrt{a+c}+c\sqrt{a+b}} \quad (1)$$

Since the inequality is symmetric, WLOG, we may assume that $a \leq b \leq c$. Then we know that $\sqrt{a+b}\leq \sqrt{a+c}\leq \sqrt{b+c}$

Then we have the following two similarly ordered sequences:

a, b, c

$\sqrt{a+b}, \sqrt{a+c}, \sqrt{b+c}$

By the rearrangement inequality, we have

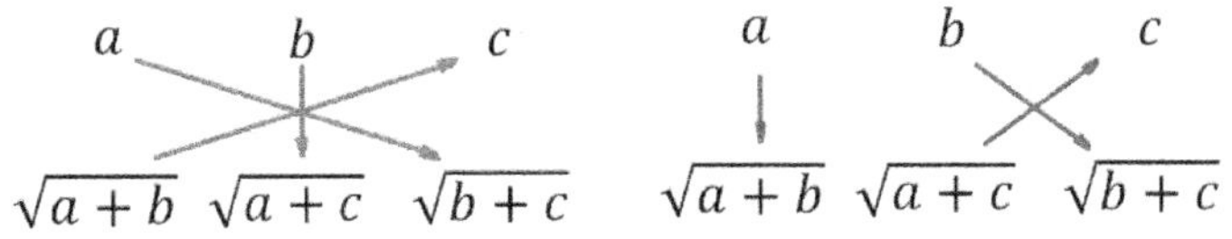

$a \quad b \quad c \qquad a \quad b \quad c$

$\sqrt{a+b} \; \sqrt{a+c} \; \sqrt{b+c} \qquad \sqrt{a+b} \; \sqrt{a+c} \; \sqrt{b+c}$

$$a\sqrt{b+c} + b\sqrt{a+c} + c\sqrt{a+b} \le c\sqrt{a+b} + b\sqrt{a+c} + a\sqrt{b+c} \qquad (2)$$

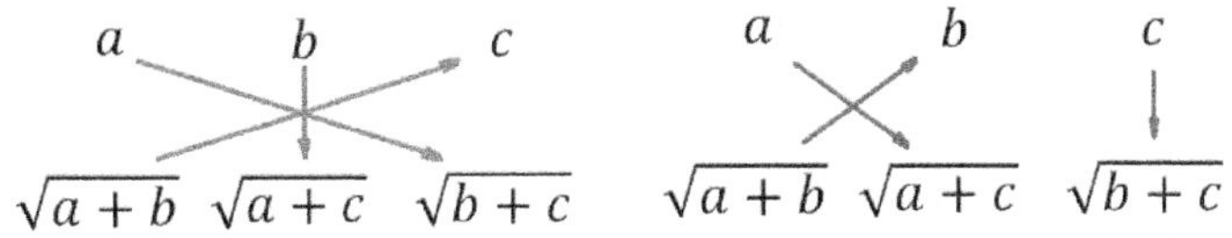

$a \quad b \quad c \qquad a \quad b \quad c$

$\sqrt{a+b} \; \sqrt{a+c} \; \sqrt{b+c} \qquad \sqrt{a+b} \; \sqrt{a+c} \; \sqrt{b+c}$

$$a\sqrt{b+c} + b\sqrt{a+c} + c\sqrt{a+b} \le b\sqrt{a+b} + a\sqrt{a+c} + c\sqrt{b+c} \qquad (3)$$

We also have

$$a\sqrt{b+c} + b\sqrt{a+c} + c\sqrt{a+b} \le a\sqrt{b+c} + b\sqrt{a+c} + c\sqrt{a+b} \qquad (4)$$

(2) + (3) + (4):

$3(a\sqrt{b+c} + b\sqrt{a+c} + c\sqrt{a+b}) \le (a+b+c)(\sqrt{a+b} + \sqrt{a+c} + \sqrt{b+c}$

Or

$a\sqrt{b+c} + b\sqrt{a+c} + c\sqrt{a+b} \le \frac{1}{3}(a+b+c)(\sqrt{a+b} + \sqrt{a+c} + \sqrt{b+c}$

$\le \frac{1}{3}(\sqrt{3[(a+b) + a + c) + (b+c)]}$

$= \frac{\sqrt{6}}{3} \qquad (5)$

Substituting (5) into (1):

$$\frac{a^2}{a\sqrt{b+c}} + \frac{b^2}{b\sqrt{c+a}} + \frac{c^2}{c\sqrt{a+b}} \ge \frac{1}{\frac{\sqrt{6}}{3}} = \sqrt{\frac{3}{2}}.$$ QED.

Problem 10. Solution:

For the following similarly ordered sequences,

a, b, c, d

d^3, c^3, b^3, a^3

by the rearrangement inequality, we have

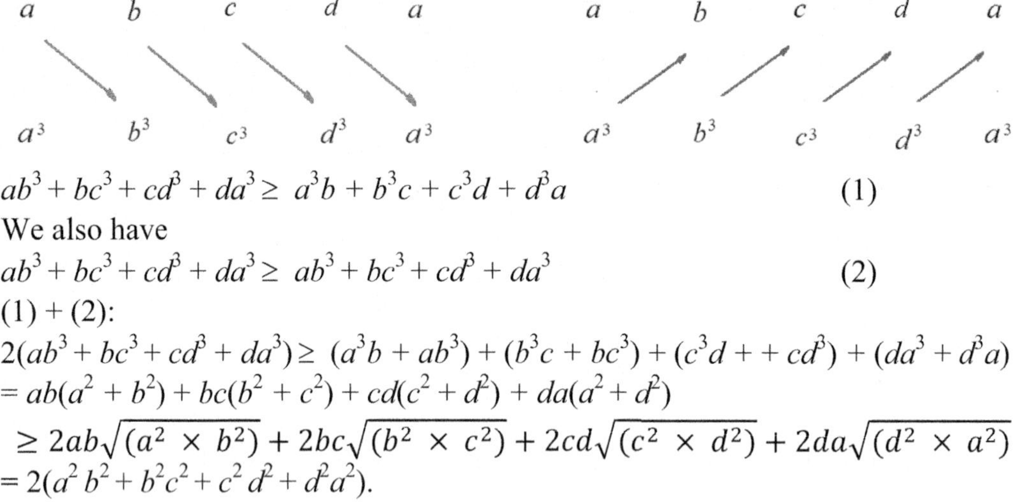

$ab^3 + bc^3 + cd^3 + da^3 \geq a^3b + b^3c + c^3d + d^3a$ (1)

We also have

$ab^3 + bc^3 + cd^3 + da^3 \geq ab^3 + bc^3 + cd^3 + da^3$ (2)

(1) + (2):

$2(ab^3 + bc^3 + cd^3 + da^3) \geq (a^3b + ab^3) + (b^3c + bc^3) + (c^3d + + cd^3) + (da^3 + d^3a)$

$= ab(a^2 + b^2) + bc(b^2 + c^2) + cd(c^2 + d^2) + da(a^2 + d^2)$

$\geq 2ab\sqrt{(a^2 \times b^2)} + 2bc\sqrt{(b^2 \times c^2)} + 2cd\sqrt{(c^2 \times d^2)} + 2da\sqrt{(d^2 \times a^2)}$

$= 2(a^2 b^2 + b^2c^2 + c^2 d^2 + d^2a^2)$.

That is, $ab^3 + bc^3 + cd^3 + da^3 \geq a^2 b^2 + b^2c^2 + c^2 d^2 + d^2a^2$.

Method 2:

By Cauchy,

$(x_1^2 + x_2^2 + x_3^2 + x_4^2) \cdot (y_1^2 + y_2^2 + y_3^2 + y_4^2) \geq (x_1y_1 + x_2y_2 + x_3y_3 + x_4y_4)^2$ (1)

Let $x_1 = b\sqrt{ab}$, $x_2 = c\sqrt{bc}$, $x_3 = d\sqrt{cd}$, $x_4 = a\sqrt{da}$,

$y_1 = a\sqrt{ab}$, $y_2 = b\sqrt{bc}$, $y_3 = c\sqrt{cd}$, $y_4 = d\sqrt{da}$.

Substituting into (1):

$[(b\sqrt{ab})^2 + (c\sqrt{bc})^2 + (d\sqrt{cd})^2 + (a\sqrt{da})^2][(a\sqrt{ab})^2 + (b\sqrt{bc})^2 + (c\sqrt{cd})^2 + (d\sqrt{da})^2]$

$\geq [(b\sqrt{ab})(a\sqrt{ab}) + (c\sqrt{bc})(b\sqrt{bc}) + (d\sqrt{cd})(c\sqrt{cd}) + (a\sqrt{da})(d\sqrt{da})]^2$

or

$(ab^3 + bc^3 + cd^3 + da^3)(a^3b + b^3c + c^3d + d^3a) \geq (a^2b^2 + b^2c^2 + c^2d^2 + d^2a^2)^2$ (2)

Then we have the following two similarly ordered sequences:

a, b, c, d

$a^3, b^3 c^3, d^3$

By the rearrangement inequality, we have

$ab^3 + bc^3 + cd^3 + da^3 \ge ad^3 + ba^3 + cb^3 + dc^3$

or $ab^3 + bc^3 + cd^3 + da^3 \ge a^3b + b^3c + c^3d + d^3a$ (3)

Multiplying (3) by $ab^3 + bc^3 + cd^3 + da^3$:

$(ab^3 + bc^3 + cd^3 + da^3)^2 \ge (ab^3 + bc^3 + cd^3 + da^3)(a^3b + b^3c + c^3d + d^3a)$ (4)

Comparing (2) and (4), we have:

$(ab^3 + bc^3 + cd^3 + da^3)^2 \ge (a^2b^2 + b^2c^2 + c^2d^2 + d^2a^2)^2$,

That is $ab^3 + bc^3 + cd^3 + da^3 \ge a^2b^2 + b^2c^2 + c^2d^2 + d^2a^2$. QED.

Problem 11. Solution:

Since the expression is a symmetric function of a, b and c, we can assume, without loss of generality, that $a \le b \le c$. $a^2 \le b^2 \le c^2$. We also see that

$$\frac{1}{2a^3 + b^3 + c^3} \ge \frac{1}{2b^3 + c^3 + a^3} \ge \frac{1}{2c^3 + a^3 + b^3}$$

Then we have the following two similarly ordered sequences:

$a^2,\ b^2,\ c^2,$

$$\frac{1}{2c^3 + a^3 + b^3}, \frac{1}{2b^3 + c^3 + a^3}, \frac{1}{2a^3 + b^3 + c^3}$$

By the rearrangement inequality,

$$\begin{matrix} a^2 & b^2 & c^2 \\ \frac{1}{2c^3+a^3+b^3} & \frac{1}{2b^3+c^3+a^3} & \frac{1}{2a^3+b^3+c^3} \end{matrix}$$

we see that $\frac{a^2}{2a^3+b^3+c^3} + \frac{b^2}{2b^3+c^3+a^3} + \frac{c^2}{2c^3+a^3+b^3}$ is the smallest value among all the rearrangements.

Now by Cauchy, $\frac{1}{a^3+b^3}+\frac{1}{a^3+c^3} \geq \frac{(1+1)^2}{2a^3+b^3+c^3}$, thus $\frac{1}{2a^3+b^3+c^3} \leq \frac{1}{4}(\frac{1}{a^3+b^3}+\frac{1}{a^3+c^3})$.

Similarly, we have $\frac{1}{2b^3+c^3+a^3} \leq \frac{1}{4}(\frac{1}{b^3+c^3}+\frac{1}{b^3+a^3})$; $\frac{1}{2c^3+a^3+b^3} \leq \frac{1}{4}(\frac{1}{c^3+a^3}+\frac{1}{a^3+b^3})$.

The left hand side of the inequality can be written as

$$\frac{a^3}{2a^3+b^3+c^3}+\frac{b^3}{2b^3+c^3+a^3}+\frac{c^3}{2c^3+a^3+b^3}$$

$$\leq \frac{1}{4}(\frac{1}{a^3+b^3}+\frac{1}{a^3+c^3}+\frac{1}{b^3+c^3}+\frac{1}{b^3+a^3}+\frac{1}{c^3+a^3})$$

$$= \frac{1}{4}(\frac{a^2+b^2}{a^3+b^3}+\frac{a^2+c^2}{a^3+c^3}+\frac{b^2+c^2}{b^3+c^3}).$$

For the similarly ordered two sequences:
$a,\ b,$
$a^2,\ b^2$
by the rearrangement inequality,

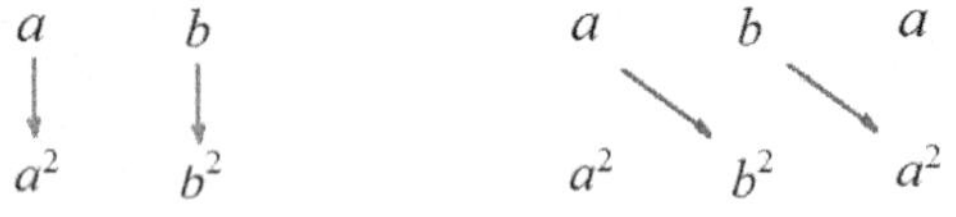

a ↓ a^2 $\quad$ b ↓ b^2 $\qquad\qquad$ $a\ \ b\ \ a$ ↘ $a^2\ \ b^2\ \ a^2$

we have
$a^3+b^3 \geq a^3+b^3$ (1)
$a^3+b^3 \geq a^2b+ab^2$ (2)

(1) + (2):
$2(a^3+b^3) \geq a^3+b^3+a^2b+ab^2 = a^3+ab^2+b^3+a^2b$
$= a(a^2+b^2)+b(b^2+a^2) = (a+b)(a^2+b^2)$.

Thus $a^3+b^3 \geq \frac{1}{2}(a+b)(a^2+b^2)$.

Similarly, we have

$$a^3 + c^3 \geq \frac{1}{2}(a + c)(a^2 + c^2)$$

$$b^3 + c^3 \geq \frac{1}{2}(b + c)(b^2 + c^2).$$

Then

$$\frac{1}{4}\left(\frac{a^2 + b^2}{a^3 + b^3} + \frac{a^2 + c^2}{a^3 + c^3} + \frac{b^2 + c^2}{b^3 + c^3}\right)$$

$$= \frac{1}{4}\left(\frac{a^2 + b^2}{\frac{1}{2}(a + b)(a^2 + b^2)} + \frac{a^2 + c^2}{\frac{1}{2}(a + c)(a^2 + c^2)} + \frac{b^2 + c^2}{\frac{1}{2}(b + c)(b^2 + c^2)}\right)$$

$$= \frac{1}{2}\left(\frac{1}{a + b} + \frac{1}{a + c} + \frac{1}{b + c}\right)$$

By AM-GM, we know that

$$a + b \geq 2\sqrt{ab}$$

$$a + c \geq 2\sqrt{ac}$$

$$c + b \geq 2\sqrt{cb}$$

Thus $\frac{1}{2}\left(\frac{1}{a+b} + \frac{1}{a+c} + \frac{1}{b+c}\right) = \frac{1}{2}\left(\frac{\sqrt{abc}}{a+b} + \frac{\sqrt{abc}}{a+c} + \frac{\sqrt{abc}}{b+c}\right)$

$\leq \frac{1}{2}\left(\frac{\sqrt{abc}}{2\sqrt{ab}} + \frac{\sqrt{abc}}{2\sqrt{ac}} + \frac{\sqrt{abc}}{2\sqrt{cb}}\right) = \frac{\sqrt{a}+\sqrt{b}+\sqrt{c}}{4}$. QED.

Problem 12. Solution:

Method 1:

By AM-GM, we have $a + b \geq 2\sqrt{ab}$. Thus $2\sqrt{ab} \leq 2ab$, or $ab \geq 1$. Thus $a + b \geq 2$.

Since the inequality is symmetric, we assume that $a \leq b$ and $b \geq 1$ and $a \leq 1$.

$$\frac{a}{a^2+b} + \frac{b}{b^2+a} \leq 1 \quad \Leftrightarrow \quad \frac{a}{a^2+b} \leq 1 - \frac{b}{b^2+a} = \frac{b^2+a-b}{b^2+a}$$

$$\Leftrightarrow \quad a(b^2 + a) \leq (a^2 + b)(b^2 + a - b)$$

$$\Leftrightarrow \quad a^2b^2 + b^3 + a^3 + ab - a^2b - b^2 - ab^2 - a^2 \geq 0$$

$$\Leftrightarrow \quad a^3 + a^2(b^2 - b - 1) - ab(b - 1) + b^2(b - 1) \geq 0$$

$$\Leftrightarrow \quad a^2[(b(b - 1) + a - 1] + b(b - 1)(b - a) \geq 0 \qquad (1)$$

We know that $b(b - 1) + a - 1 \geq b - 1 + a - 1 = a + b - 2 \geq 0$.

Thus every term on the left hand side of (1) is nonnegative. Therefore (1) is true. QED.

Method 2:

For the following inequality:

$\frac{a}{b^2+a}+\frac{b}{a^2+b}\le 1 \quad\Leftrightarrow\quad \frac{a}{b^2+a}\le 1-\frac{b}{a^2+b}=\frac{a^2}{a^2+b} \quad\Leftrightarrow\quad \frac{1}{b^2+a}\le\frac{a}{a^2+b}$

$\Leftrightarrow \quad a^2+b\le a(b^2+a) \Leftrightarrow \quad ab\ge 1$, which is true.

Thus $\frac{a}{b^2+a}+\frac{b}{a^2+b}\le 1$.

Since the inequality is symmetric, WLOG, we assume that $a\le b$.

Then we have $b^2+a\ge a^2+b$.

We have the following similarly ordered sequences:

a, b

$\frac{1}{b^2+a}, \frac{1}{a^2+b}$

By rearrangement inequality, we have

$$\begin{matrix} a & b \\ \frac{1}{b^2+a} & \frac{1}{a^2+b} \end{matrix} \;(\text{crossed}) \le \begin{matrix} a & b \\ \downarrow & \downarrow \\ \frac{1}{b^2+a} & \frac{1}{a^2+b} \end{matrix}$$

or $\begin{bmatrix} a & b \\ \frac{1}{a^2+b} & \frac{1}{b^2+a} \end{bmatrix}\le\begin{bmatrix} a & b \\ \frac{1}{b^2+a} & \frac{1}{a^2+b} \end{bmatrix}$.

That is $\frac{a}{a^2+b}+\frac{b}{b^2+a}\le\frac{a}{b^2+a}+\frac{b}{a^2+b}$.

Since we already prove that $\frac{a}{b^2+a}+\frac{b}{a^2+b}\le 1$, $\frac{a}{a^2+b}+\frac{b}{b^2+a}\le\frac{a}{b^2+a}+\frac{b}{a^2+b}\le 1$.

QED.

Chapter 7 Solving Math Olympiad Problems

Example 1. (1969 Canadian Math Olympiad) Let c be the length of the hypotenuse of a right angle triangle whose other two sides have lengths a and b. Prove that $a + b \le \sqrt{2}c$. When does the equality hold?

Solution:

Method 1 (official solution):

Since $a > 0$, $b > 0$ and $(a - b)^2 \ge 0$, we have $a^2 + b^2 \ge 2ab$.

$2(a^2 + b^2) \ge 2ab + a^2 + b^2 = (a + b)^2$, $\sqrt{2}\sqrt{(a^2+b^2)} \ge a + b$

Since $c^2 = a^2+b^2$, $\sqrt{2}c \ge a + b$ with equality if and only if $(a - b)^2 = 0$, i.e. $a= b$.

Method 2.

We have the following two similarly ordered sequences:

a, b

a, b

By the rearrangement inequality, we have

$$\begin{matrix} a & b \\ \downarrow & \downarrow \\ a & b \end{matrix} \qquad \begin{matrix} a & & b \\ & \times & \\ a & & b \end{matrix}$$

$a \cdot a + b \cdot b = a^2 + b^2 \ge a \cdot b + a \cdot b = 2ab \Leftrightarrow$

$a^2 + b^2 + a^2 + b^2 \ge 2ab + a^2 + b^2 \Leftrightarrow$

$2(a^2 + b^2) \ge (a + b)^2 \Leftrightarrow$

$2c^2 \ge (a + b)^2 \Leftrightarrow$

$a + b \le \sqrt{2}c.$

Equality of this inequality occurs if and only if $a = b$.

Example 2. (2002 Canadian Mathematical Olympiad) Prove that for all positive real numbers *a, b,* and *c*, $\frac{a^3}{bc}+\frac{b^3}{ca}+\frac{c^3}{ab}\geq a+b+c$, and determine when equality occurs.

Proof:
Each of the inequalities used in the solutions below has the property that equality holds if and only if $a = b = c$. Thus, equality holds for the given inequality if and only if $a = b = c$.

There are 3 official solutions to this problem. We provide the solution 4 using the rearrangement inequality and solution 5 using AM-GM.

Method 1:
Note that $a^4 + b^4 + c^4 = (a^4 + b^4)/2 + (b^4 + c^4)/2 + (c^4 + a^4)/2$.

Applying the arithmetic-geometric mean inequality to each term, we see that the right side is greater than or equal to $a^2b^2 + b^2c^2 + c^2a^2$. We can rewrite this as $a^2(b^2 + c^2)/2 + b^2(c^2 + a^2)/2 + c^2(a^2 + b^2)/2$.

Applying the arithmetic mean-geometric mean inequality again we obtain $a^4 + b^4 + c^4 \geq a^2bc + b^2ca + c^2ab$. Dividing both sides by *abc* (which is positive) the result follows.

Method 2:
Notice the inequality is homogeneous. That is, if *a, b, c* are replaced by *ka, kb, kc,* $k > 0$ we get the original inequality. Thus we can assume, without loss of generality, that $abc = 1$. Then $a^3/bc + b^3/ca + c^3/ab = abc\,(a^3/bc + b^3/ca + c^3/ab) = a^4 + b^4 + c^4$. So we need prove that $a^4 + b^4 + c^4 \geq a + b + c$. By the Power Mean Inequality, $(a^4 + b^4 + c^4)/3 \geq [(a + b + c)/3]^4$, so $a^4 + b^4 + c^4 \geq (a + b + c) \cdot (a + b + c)^3 /27$. By the arithmetic mean-geometric mean inequality,

$\frac{a+b+c}{3} \geq \sqrt[3]{abc} = 1$, so $a + b + c \geq 3$. Hence,

$$a^4+b^4+c^4 \geq (a+b+c)\cdot\frac{(a+b+c)^3}{27} \geq (a+b+c)\cdot\frac{(3)^3}{27} = a+b+c$$

Method 3:
Rather than using the Power-Mean inequality to prove $a^4 + b^4 + c^4 \geq a + b + c$ in Proof 2, the Cauchy inequality can be used twice:
$(a^4 + b^4 + c^4)(1^2 + 1^2 + 1^2) \geq (a^2 + b^2 + c^2)^2$
$(a^2 + b^2 + c^2)(1^2 + 1^2 + 1^2) \geq (a + b + c)^2$

So $\frac{a^4+b^4+c^4}{3} \geq \frac{(a^2+b^2+c^2)^2}{9} \geq \frac{(a+b+c)^4}{81}$
Continue as in Proof 2.

Method 4:
Since the inequality is symmetric, WLOG, we may assume that $a \leq b \leq c$. Then we know that $a^3 \leq b^3 \leq c^3$.
Then we have the following two similarly ordered sequences:
a^3, b^3, c^3.
$\frac{1}{bc}, \frac{1}{ac}, \frac{1}{ab}$

By the rearrangement inequality, we have

$$\begin{array}{ccc} a^3 & b^3 & c^3 \\ \downarrow & \downarrow & \downarrow \\ \frac{1}{bc} & \frac{1}{ac} & \frac{1}{ab} \end{array} \qquad \begin{array}{ccccccc} a^3 & & b^3 & & c^3 & & a^3 \\ & \searrow & & \searrow & & \searrow & \\ \frac{1}{bc} & & \frac{1}{ac} & & \frac{1}{ab} & & \frac{1}{bc} \end{array}$$

$$\frac{a^3}{bc} + \frac{b^3}{ca} + \frac{c^3}{ab} \geq \frac{a^3}{ac} + \frac{b^3}{ab} + \frac{c^3}{bc} = \frac{a^2}{c} + \frac{b^2}{a} + \frac{c^2}{b} \qquad (1)$$

Then we have the following two similarly ordered sequences:
a^2, b^2, c^2.
$\frac{1}{c}, \frac{1}{b}, \frac{1}{a}$

By the rearrangement inequality, we have

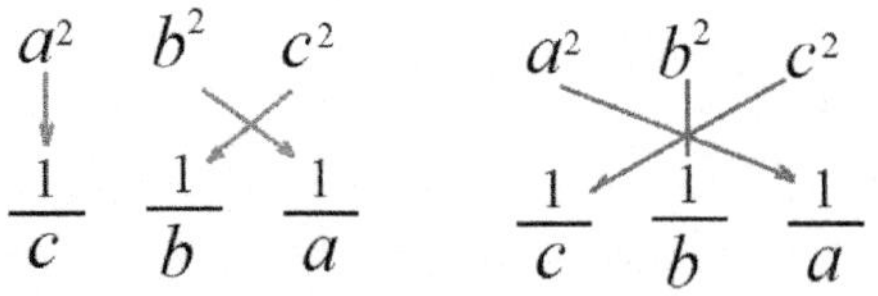

$$\begin{array}{ccc} a^2 & b^2 & c^2 \\ \downarrow & \times & \\ \frac{1}{c} & \frac{1}{b} & \frac{1}{a} \end{array} \qquad \begin{array}{ccc} a^2 & b^2 & c^2 \\ & \text{(crossed)} & \\ \frac{1}{c} & \frac{1}{b} & \frac{1}{a} \end{array}$$

$$\frac{a^2}{c}+\frac{b^2}{a}+\frac{c^2}{b}\geq \frac{a^2}{a}+\frac{c^2}{c}+\frac{b^2}{b}=a+b+c$$

$$\frac{a^3}{bc}+\frac{b^3}{ca}+\frac{c^3}{ab}\geq a+b+c,$$

Method 5:

From AM-GM, we have

$$\frac{a^3}{bc}+b+c\geq 3\sqrt[3]{\frac{a^3}{bc}\cdot b\cdot c}=3a \qquad (1)$$

Similarly,

$$\frac{b^3}{ac}+a+c\geq 3\sqrt[3]{\frac{b^3}{ac}\cdot a\cdot c}=3b \qquad (2)$$

$$\frac{c^3}{ab}+a+b\geq 3\sqrt[3]{\frac{c^3}{ab}\cdot a\cdot b}=3c \qquad (3)$$

(1) + (2) + (3):

$$\frac{a^3}{bc}+\frac{b^3}{ac}+\frac{c^3}{ab}+2(a+b+c)\geq 3(a+b+c)$$

$$\frac{a^3}{bc}+\frac{b^3}{ca}+\frac{c^3}{ab}\geq a+b+c\,.$$

Example 3. (2004 Hong Kong IMO Team Training Problem) Prove that for all positive real numbers *a, b,* and *c*, $\frac{a^4}{bc}+\frac{b^4}{ca}+\frac{c^4}{ab}\geq a^2+b^2+c^2$.

Proof:

Since the inequality is symmetric, WLOG, we may assume that $a\leq b\leq c$. Then we know that $a^4\leq b^4\leq c^4$.

Then we have the following two similarly ordered sequences:

a^4, b^4, c^4.

$\frac{1}{bc}, \frac{1}{ac}, \frac{1}{ab}$

By the rearrangement inequality, we have

$a^4 \quad b^4 \quad c^4 \qquad\qquad a^4 \quad b^4 \quad c^4 \quad a^4$

$\frac{1}{bc} \quad \frac{1}{ac} \quad \frac{1}{ab} \qquad\qquad \frac{1}{bc} \quad \frac{1}{ac} \quad \frac{1}{ab} \quad \frac{1}{bc}$

$$\frac{a^4}{bc}+\frac{b^4}{ca}+\frac{c^4}{ab} \ge \frac{a^4}{ac}+\frac{b^4}{ab}+\frac{c^4}{bc} = \frac{a^3}{c}+\frac{b^3}{a}+\frac{c^3}{b} \qquad (1)$$

Then we have the following two similarly ordered sequences:

a^3, b^3, c^3.

$\frac{1}{c}, \frac{1}{b}, \frac{1}{a}$

By the rearrangement inequality, we have

$a^3 \quad b^3 \quad c^3 \qquad\qquad a^3 \quad b^3 \quad c^3$

$\frac{1}{c} \quad \frac{1}{b} \quad \frac{1}{a} \qquad\qquad \frac{1}{c} \quad \frac{1}{b} \quad \frac{1}{a}$

$$\frac{a^3}{c}+\frac{b^3}{a}+\frac{c^3}{b} \ge \frac{a^3}{a}+\frac{c^3}{c}+\frac{b^3}{b} = a^2+b^2+c^2$$

Example 4. (1992 Canadian Math Olympiad) For $x, y, z \ge 0$, establish the inequality $x(x-z)^2 + y(y-z)^2 \ge (x-z)(y-z)(x+y-z)$ and determine when equality holds.

Solution:

Method 1:

The given inequality is equivalent to the following inequality:

$x(x-z)^2 + y(y-z)^2 - (x-z)(y-z)(x+y-z) \ge 0$

We see that

$x(x-z)^2 + y(y-z)^2 - (x-z)(y-z)(x+y-z)$

$= x^3 - 2x^2z - xz^2 + y^3 - 2y^2z + yz^2 - x^2y - xy^2 + xyz + x^2z + xyz - xz^2 + xyx + y^2z$
$- yz^2 - z^2 (x + y - z)$
$= (x^3 - x^2z - x^2y) + (y^3 - y^2z - xy^2) + 3xyz - z^2(x + y - z)$
$= -x^2 (y + z - x) - y^2(x + z - y) - z^2(x + y - z) + 3xyz.$

The given inequality is equivalent to the following inequality:
$-x^2 (y + z - x) - y^2(x + z - y) - z^2(x + y - z) + 3xyz \ge 0$
or $x^2 (y + z - x) + y^2(x + z - y) + z^2(x + y - z) \le 3xyz$

Since the expression is a symmetric function of x, y and z, we can assume, without loss of generality, that $x \le y \le z$.

We see that $z(y + x - z) - y(z + x - y) = zy + zx - z^2 - yz - yx + y^2$
$= x(z - y) + (y^2 - z^2) = (y - z)(y + z - x) \le 0.$

Similarly we have $x(z + y - x) \ge y(x + z - y)$.

Then we have the following two similarly ordered sequences:
x, y, z
$z(x + y - z), y(x + z - y), x(y + z - x),$

By the rearrangement inequality, we have

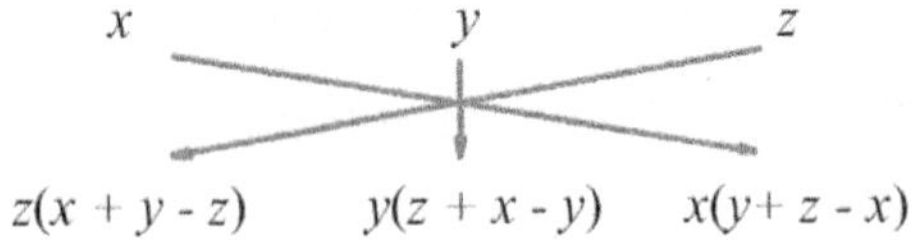

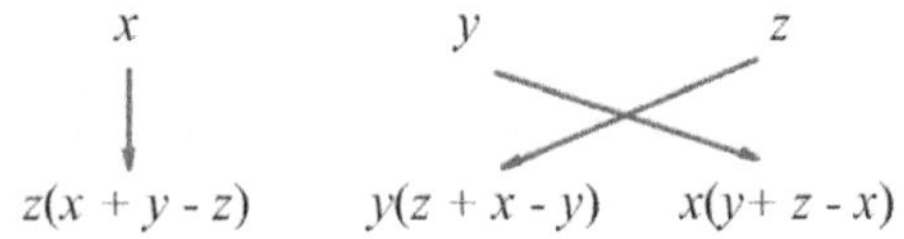

x y z x y z

$z(x + y - z)$ $y(z + x - y)$ $x(y + z - x)$ $z(x + y - z)$ $y(z + x - y)$ $x(y + z - x)$

$x^2 (y + z - x) + y^2(x + z - y) + z^2(x + y - z)$
$\le xz(y + z - x) + yx(x + z - y) + zx(x + y - z)$ (1)
$= 3xyz + xy(y - x) + yz(z - y) + xz(x - z)$

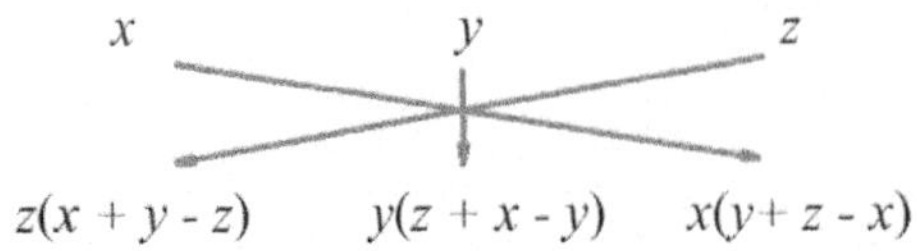

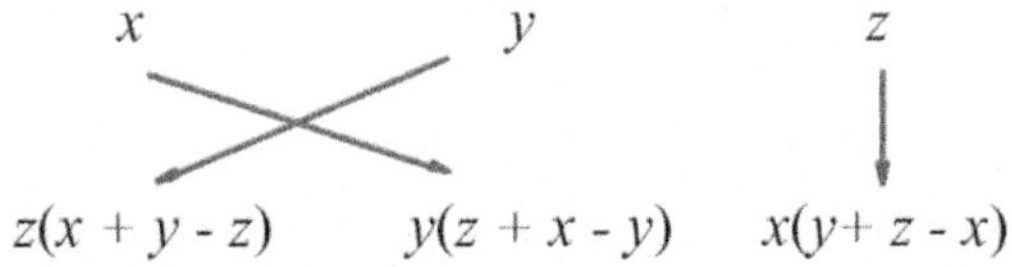

x y z x y z

$z(x + y - z)$ $y(z + x - y)$ $x(y + z - x)$ $z(x + y - z)$ $y(z + x - y)$ $x(y + z - x)$

$x^2(y+z-x)+y^2(x+z-y)+z^2(x+y-z)$
$\le yz(y+z-x)+xy(x+z-y)+zx(x+y-z)$ (2)
$= 3xyz - xy(y-x) - yz(z-y) - xz(x-z)$

(1) + (2):
$2[x^2(y+z-x)+y^2(x+z-y)+z^2(x+y-z)] \le 6xyz \quad \Rightarrow$
$x^2(y+z-x)+y^2(x+z-y)+z^2(x+y-z) \le 3xyz$

The equality holds when $x(y+z-x) = y(x+z-y) = z(x+y-z)$, or $x = y = z$. That is, $x = z,\ y = 0$; or $y = z,\ x = 0$; or $x = y,\ z = 0$; or $x = y = z$.

Method 2:
We do the following replacements:
$x \Rightarrow y$, and we get $y(y-z)^2 + x(x-z)^2 \ge (y-z)(x-z)(y+x-z)$

We see that the new expression is the same as the given one. So it is symmetric.

Since the inequality is a symmetric function of x, y and z, we can assume, without loss of generality, that $x \le z \le y$.

We see that $x(x-z)^2 + y(y-z)^2 \ge 0 \ge (x-z)(y-z)(x+y-z)$.

The equality holds when $x(y+z-x) = y(x+z-y) = z(x+y-z)$, or $x = y = z$.

That is, $x = z,\ y = 0$; or $y = z,\ x = 0$; or $x = y,\ z = 0$; or $x = y = z$.

Example 5. (1995 IMO) If a, b, $c > 0$ and $abc = 1$, show that

$$\frac{1}{a^3(b+c)} + \frac{1}{b^3(a+c)} + \frac{1}{c^3(a+b)} \ge \frac{3}{2}.$$

Solution:
Method 1:
Let $x = \frac{1}{a}$, $y = \frac{1}{b}$, $z = \frac{1}{c}$. Then we have $xyz = 1$. $x + y + z \ge 3$.

The original inequality can be written as

$$\frac{x^2}{y+z}+\frac{y^2}{z+x}+\frac{z^2}{x+y}\ge\frac{3}{2}.$$

By the symmetrical property, we assume that $x\le y\le z$

Then we have $x^2\le y^2\le z^2$ and $\frac{1}{y+z}\le\frac{1}{z+x}\le\frac{1}{x+y}$

For the following similarly ordered sequences,

x^2,y^2,z^2

$\frac{1}{y+z},\frac{1}{z+x},\frac{1}{x+y}$

based on the rearrangement inequality,

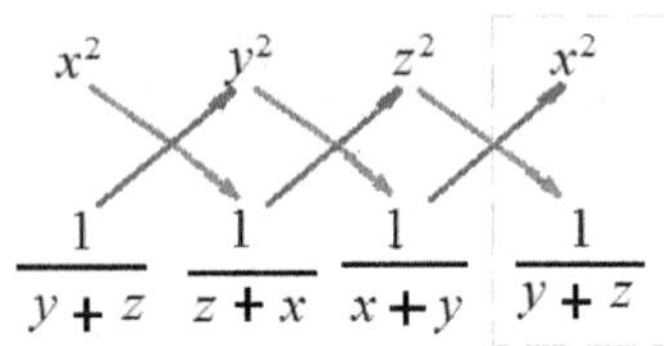

So

$$\frac{x^2}{y+z}+\frac{y^2}{z+x}+\frac{z^2}{x+y}\ge\frac{x^2}{z+x}+\frac{y^2}{x+y}+\frac{z^2}{y+z}\qquad(1)$$

$$\frac{x^2}{y+z}+\frac{y^2}{z+x}+\frac{z^2}{x+y}\ge\frac{y^2}{y+z}+\frac{z^2}{z+x}+\frac{x^2}{x+y}\qquad(2)$$

(1) + (2): $2(\frac{x^2}{y+z}+\frac{y^2}{z+x}+\frac{z^2}{x+y})\ge\frac{x^2+z^2}{z+x}+\frac{y^2+x^2}{x+y}+\frac{z^2+y^2}{y+z}$

Since $\frac{x^2+z^2}{z+x}+\frac{y^2+x^2}{x+y}+\frac{z^2+y^2}{y+z}\ge\frac{x+z}{2}+\frac{y+x}{2}+\frac{z+y}{2}=x+y+z\ge 3$

We get $\frac{x^2}{y+z}+\frac{y^2}{z+x}+\frac{z^2}{x+y}\geq\frac{3}{2}$.

Method 2:

$$\frac{1}{a^3(b+c)}+\frac{1}{b^3(a+c)}+\frac{1}{c^3(a+b)}$$

$$=\frac{(abc)^3}{a^3(b+c)}+\frac{(abc)^3}{b^3(a+c)}+\frac{(abc)^3}{c^3(a+b)}$$

$$=\frac{(bc)^2}{a(b+c)}+\frac{(ac)^2}{b(a+c)}+\frac{(ab)^2}{c(a+b)}$$

$$=\frac{bc}{a(b+c)}\cdot bc+\frac{ac}{b(a+c)}\cdot ac+\frac{ab}{c(a+b)}\cdot ab$$

By the symmetrical property, we assume that $a\leq b\leq c$. So we can have $ab\leq ac$ $\leq bc$, $ab+ac\leq ab+bc\leq ac+bc$, and $\frac{1}{c(a+b)}\leq\frac{1}{b(b+c)}\leq\frac{1}{a(b+c)}$.

For the following similarly ordered sequences,

$ab, ac, bc,$

$ab, ac, bc,$

$$\frac{1}{c(a+b)},\frac{1}{b(b+c)},\frac{1}{a(b+c)}.$$

based on the rearrangement inequality,

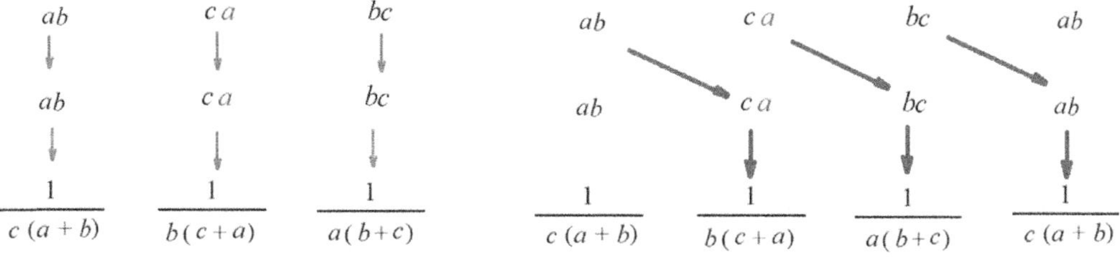

we have

$$\frac{ab}{c(a+b)}\cdot ab+\frac{bc}{a(b+c)}\cdot bc+\frac{ac}{b(a+c)}\cdot ac$$
$$\geq \frac{ab}{c(a+b)}\cdot bc+\frac{ca}{b(c+a)}\cdot ab+\frac{bc}{a(b+c)}\cdot ca \qquad (1)$$

and

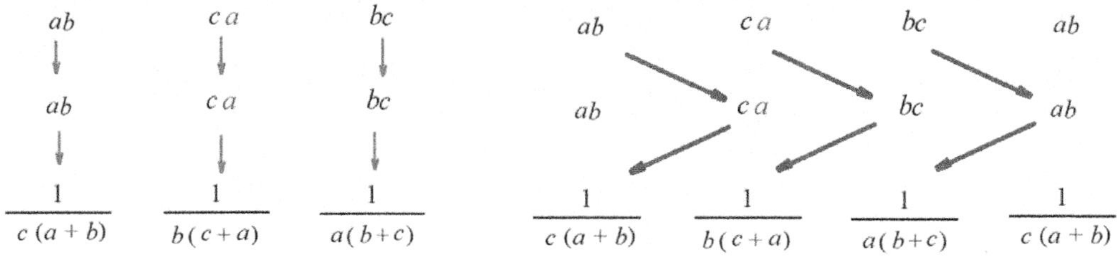

ab	ca	bc
↓	↓	↓
ab	ca	bc
↓	↓	↓
$\frac{1}{c(a+b)}$	$\frac{1}{b(c+a)}$	$\frac{1}{a(b+c)}$

ab	ca	bc	ab
ab	ca	bc	ab
$\frac{1}{c(a+b)}$	$\frac{1}{b(c+a)}$	$\frac{1}{a(b+c)}$	$\frac{1}{c(a+b)}$

$$\frac{ab}{c(a+b)}\cdot ab+\frac{bc}{a(b+c)}\cdot bc+\frac{ac}{b(a+c)}\cdot ac$$
$$\geq \frac{ab}{c(a+b)}\cdot ca+\frac{ca}{b(c+a)}\cdot bc+\frac{bc}{a(b+c)}\cdot ab \qquad (2)$$

(1) + (2):

$$2[\frac{ab}{c(a+b)}\cdot ab+\frac{bc}{a(b+c)}\cdot bc+\frac{ac}{b(a+c)}\cdot ac]$$
$$\geq \frac{ab}{c(a+b)}\cdot bc+\frac{ca}{b(c+a)}\cdot ab+\frac{bc}{a(b+c)}\cdot ca$$
$$+\frac{ab}{c(a+b)}\cdot ca+\frac{ca}{b(c+a)}\cdot bc+\frac{bc}{a(b+c)}\cdot ab$$
$$=ab+bc+ca\geq 3\sqrt[3]{(abc)^2}=3.$$

Thus $\frac{ab}{c(a+b)}\cdot ab+\frac{bc}{a(b+c)}\cdot bc+\frac{ac}{b(a+c)}\cdot ac\geq \frac{3}{2}$.

Example 6. (2000 Poland Math Olympiad) Show that when a, b and c are real numbers with $a + b + c = 1$, $a^2 + b^2 + c^2 + 2\sqrt{3abc} \leq 1$.

Proof:

For the following similarly ordered sequences,

ab, *ac*, *bc*

ab, *ac*, *bc*

By the rearrangement inequality, we have

ab	ac	bc		ab	ac	bc	ab
↓	↓	↓		╲	╲	╲	
ab	ac	bc		ab	ac	bc	ab

$a^2b^2 + b^2c^2 + c^2a^2 \geq ab \cdot ac + ac \cdot bc + bc \cdot ab = abc\,(a + c + b)$.

Since $(ab + bc + ab)^2 \geq 3(a^2b^2 + b^2c^2a + c^2a^2) \geq 3abc\,(a + c + b)$.

$ab + bc + ca \geq \sqrt{3abc\,(a + c + b)}$

$a^2 + b^2 + c^2 + 2(ab + bc + ab) \geq a^2 + b^2 + c^2 + 2\sqrt{3abc\,(a + c + b)}$

That is $(a + b + c)^2 \geq a^2 + b^2 + c^2 + 2\sqrt{3abc\,(a + c + b)}$

Since $a + b + c = 1$, the above inequality can be written as

$a^2 + b^2 + c^2 + 2\sqrt{3abc} \leq 1$.

Method 2:

Note that

$a^2b^2 + b^2c^2 \geq 2ab^2c$

$b^2c^2 + b^2a^2 \geq 2acb^2$

$b^2a^2 + a^2c^2 \geq 2a^2bc$

Thus we have: $a^2b^2 + b^2c^2 + c^2a^2 \geq a^2bc + ab^2c + abc^2$.

So $(ab + bc + ca)^2 \geq 3(a^2bc + ab^2c + abc^2) = 3abc\,(a + b + c)$.

We know that

$a^2 + b^2 + c^2 + 2(ab + bc + ca) \geq a^2 + b^2 + c^2 + 2\sqrt{3abc(a + b + c)}$.

Since $a + b + c = 1$, the above inequality can be written as

$a^2 + b^2 + c^2 + 2\sqrt{3abc} \leq 1$.

Example 7. (1967 IMO Longlist) a, b, and c are positive real numbers. Show $\frac{a^8+b^8+c^8}{a^3b^3c^3} \ge \frac{1}{a}+\frac{1}{b}+\frac{1}{c}$.

Solution:

Since the inequality is symmetric, WLOG, we may assume that $a \le b \le c$. Then we know that $a^5 \le b^5 \le c^5$, $\frac{1}{b^3c^3} \le \frac{1}{a^3c^3} \le \frac{1}{a^3b^3}$.

Then we have the following two similarly ordered sequences:

a^5, b^5, c^5.

$\frac{1}{b^3c^3}, \frac{1}{a^3c^3}, \frac{1}{a^3b^3}$

$$\begin{matrix} a^5 & b^5 & c^5 \\ \downarrow & \downarrow & \downarrow \\ \frac{1}{b^3c^3} & \frac{1}{a^3c^3} & \frac{1}{a^3b^3} \end{matrix} \qquad \begin{matrix} a^5 & & b^5 & & c^5 & & a^5 \\ & \searrow & & \searrow & & \searrow & \\ \frac{1}{b^3c^3} & & \frac{1}{a^3c^3} & & \frac{1}{a^3b^3} & & \frac{1}{b^3c^3} \end{matrix}$$

$$\frac{a^8+b^8+c^8}{a^3b^3c^3} = \frac{a^5}{b^3c^3}+\frac{b^5}{a^3c^3}+\frac{c^5}{a^3b^3} \ge \frac{a^5}{a^3c^3}+\frac{b^5}{a^3b^3}+\frac{c^5}{b^3c^3} = \frac{a^2}{c^3}+\frac{b^2}{a^3}+\frac{c^2}{b^3}$$

Now we use the following two similarly ordered sequences:

a^2, b^2, c^2.

$\frac{1}{c^3}, \frac{1}{b^3}, \frac{1}{a^3}$

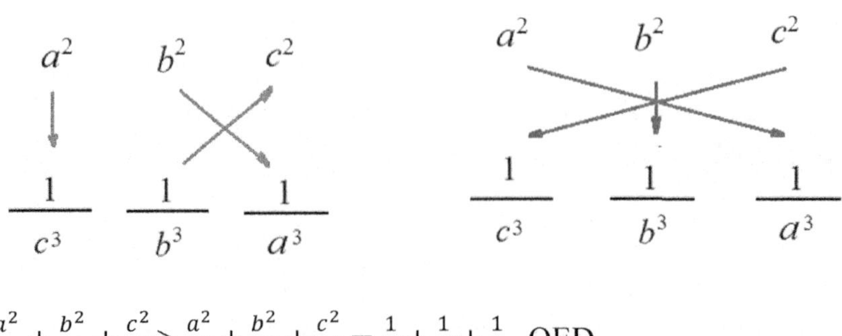

$$\frac{a^2}{c^3}+\frac{b^2}{a^3}+\frac{c^2}{b^3} \ge \frac{a^2}{a^3}+\frac{b^2}{b^3}+\frac{c^2}{c^3} = \frac{1}{a}+\frac{1}{b}+\frac{1}{c}.$$ QED.

Example 8. (1994 China MO Team Training) Let $0 \le a \le b \le c \le d \le e$ and $a + b + c + d + e = 1$. Prove that $ad + dc + cb + be + ea \le \frac{1}{5}$.

Solution:

Method 1:

Since $a \le b \le c \le d \le e$, we have $a + b \le a + c \le b + d \le c + e \le d + e$.

Then we have the following two similarly ordered sequences:

$a,\ b, c, d, e$

$a + b, a + c, b + d, c + e, d + e$

By the rearrangement inequality, we have

$a \quad b \quad c \quad d \quad e \qquad a \quad b \quad c \quad d \quad e$

$a + b \quad a + c \quad b + d \quad c + e \quad d + e \qquad a + b \quad a + c \quad b + d \quad c + e \quad d + e$

$e(a + b) + d(a + c) + c(b + d) + b(c + e) + a(d + e) \le a(a + b) + b(a + c) + c(b + d) + d(c + e) + e(d + e)$.

$2(ad + dc + cb + be + ea)$

$\le a(a + b) + b(a + c) + c(b + d) + d(c + e) + e(d + e)$ (1)

Similarly, we have $2(ad + dc + cb + be + ea)$

$\le b(a + b) + c(a + c) + d(b + d) + e(c + e) + a(d + e)$ (2)

$\le c(a + b) + d(a + c) + e(b + d) + a(c + e) + b(d + e)$ (3)

$\le d(a + b) + e(a + c) + a(b + d) + b(c + e) + c(d + e)$ (4)

$\le e(a + b) + a(a + c) + b(b + d) + c(c + e) + d(d + e)$ (5)

(1) + (2) + (3) + (4) + (5):

$10(ad + dc + cb + be + ea)$

$\le (a + b + c + d + e)(a + b + a + c + b + d + c + e + d + e)$

$\le 2(a + b + c + d + e)\ (a + b + c + d + e) = 2$.

Thus $ad + dc + cb + be + ea \le \frac{2}{10} = \frac{1}{5}$.

Method 2:
Since $a \le b \le c \le d \le e$, we have $a + b \le a + c \le b + d \le c + e \le d + e$.

Then we have the following two similarly ordered sequences:
a, b, c, d, e
$a + b, a + c, b + d, c + e, d + e$

By Chebyshev inequality, we have
$e(a + b) + d(a + c) + c(b + d) + b(c + e) + a(d + e)$
$\le \frac{1}{5}(a + b + c + d + e)[(a + b + a + c + b + d + c + e + d + e)]$
$= \frac{2}{5}(a + b + c + d + e)^2 = \frac{2}{5}$.
Thus $2(ad + dc + cb + be + ea)$
$\le \frac{2}{5}$ and $ad + dc + cb + be + ea \le \frac{1}{5}$.

Example 9. (1998 Irish Mathematical Olympiad) Prove that if a, b, c are positive real numbers, then $\frac{9}{a+b+c} \le 2\left(\frac{1}{a+b} + \frac{1}{b+c} + \frac{1}{c+a}\right)$.

Solution:
The given inequality can be written as
$$\frac{a+b+c}{a+b} + \frac{a+b+c}{b+c} + \frac{a+b+c}{c+a} \ge \frac{9}{2}$$
or $3 + \frac{c}{a+b} + \frac{a}{b+c} + \frac{b}{c+a} \ge \frac{9}{2}$ or $\frac{c}{a+b} + \frac{a}{b+c} + \frac{b}{c+a} \ge \frac{3}{2}$

Since the inequality is symmetric, WLOG, we may assume that $a \le b \le c$ and $\frac{1}{bc} \le \frac{1}{ac} \le \frac{1}{ab}$.

Then we have the following two similarly ordered sequences:
a, b, c
$\frac{1}{b+c}, \frac{1}{a+c}, \frac{1}{a+b}$

By the rearrangement inequality, we have

$$\begin{array}{ccc} a & b & c \\ \downarrow & \downarrow & \downarrow \\ \frac{1}{b+c} & \frac{1}{c+a} & \frac{1}{a+b} \end{array} \qquad \begin{array}{ccccccc} a & & b & & c & & a \\ & \searrow & & \searrow & & \searrow & \\ \frac{1}{b+c} & & \frac{1}{c+a} & & \frac{1}{a+b} & & \frac{1}{b+c} \end{array}$$

$$\frac{a}{b+c}+\frac{b}{c+a}+\frac{c}{a+b} \ge \frac{a}{a+c}+\frac{b}{a+b}+\frac{c}{b+c} \qquad (1)$$

$$\begin{array}{ccc} a & b & c \\ \downarrow & \downarrow & \downarrow \\ \frac{1}{b+c} & \frac{1}{c+a} & \frac{1}{a+b} \end{array} \qquad \begin{array}{ccccccc} a & & b & & c & & a \\ & \nearrow & & \nearrow & & \nearrow & \\ \frac{1}{b+c} & & \frac{1}{c+a} & & \frac{1}{a+b} & & \frac{1}{b+c} \end{array}$$

$$\frac{a}{b+c}+\frac{b}{c+a}+\frac{c}{a+b} \ge \frac{c}{a+c}+\frac{a}{a+b}+\frac{b}{b+c} \qquad (2)$$

(1) + (2): $2\left(\frac{a}{b+c}+\frac{b}{a+c}+\frac{c}{a+b}\right) \ge \frac{a+c}{a+c}+\frac{b+a}{a+b}+\frac{c+b}{b+c}=3$

Thus $\frac{c}{a+b}+\frac{a}{b+c}+\frac{b}{c+a} \ge \frac{3}{2}$.

Example 10. (IMO, 1964) Suppose that a, b, c are the lengths of the sides of a triangle. Prove that $a^2(b+c-a)+b^2(a+c-b)+c^2(a+b-c) \le 3abc$.

Solution:

Since the expression is a symmetric function of a, b and c, we can assume, without loss of generality, that $a \le b \le c$.

We see that

$$b(a+c-b) \le a(b+c-a) \quad \Leftrightarrow \quad ba+bc-b^2 \le ab+ac-a^2$$
$$\Leftrightarrow \quad bc-b^2 \le ac-a^2 \quad \Leftrightarrow \quad bc-ac \le b^2-a^2$$
$$\Leftrightarrow \quad c(b-a) \le (b-a)(b+a) \quad \Leftrightarrow \quad (b-a)\,[c-(a+b)] \le 0$$

Similarly, we have $c(a+b-c) \le b(a+c-b) \le a(b+c-a)$.

Then we have the following two similarly ordered sequences:

a, $\qquad b$, $\qquad c$

$a(c-a+b),(a-b+c),c(b-c+a)$

By the rearrangement inequality

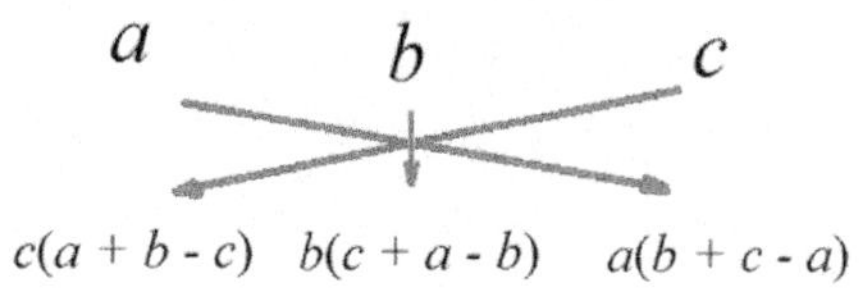

$a \quad b \quad c$

$c(a+b-c) \quad b(c+a-b) \quad a(b+c-a)$

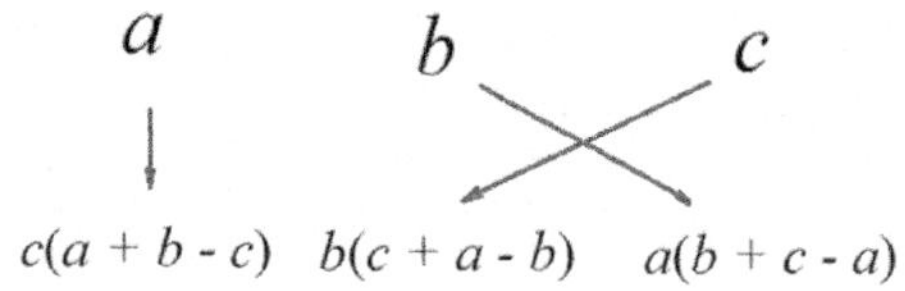

$a \quad b \quad c$

$c(a+b-c) \quad b(c+a-b) \quad a(b+c-a)$

$$a\cdot a(b+c-a)+b\cdot b(c+a-b)+c\cdot c(a+b-c)$$
$$\le a\cdot c(a+b-c)+b\cdot a(b+c-a)+c\cdot b(c+a-b) \qquad (1)$$

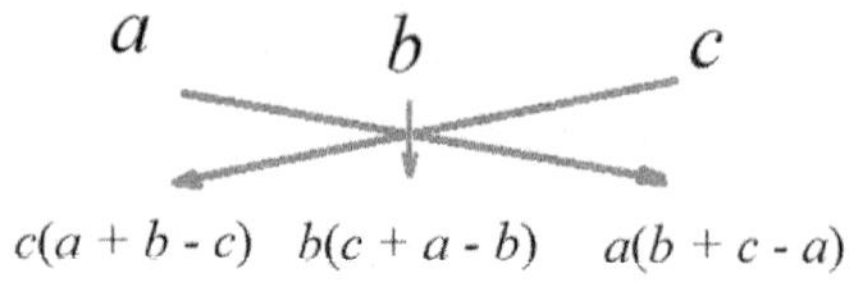

$a \quad b \quad c$

$c(a+b-c) \quad b(c+a-b) \quad a(b+c-a)$

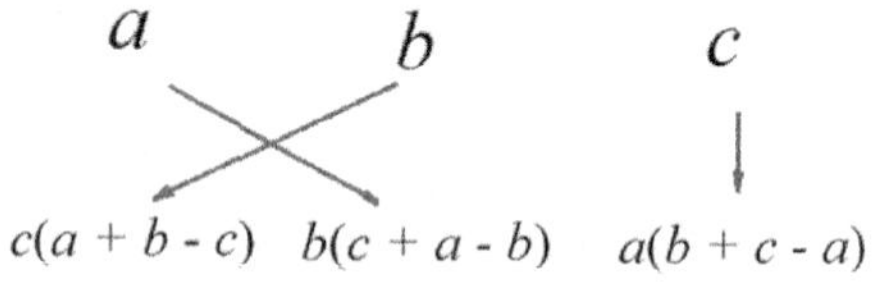

$a \quad b \quad c$

$c(a+b-c) \quad b(c+a-b) \quad a(b+c-a)$

$$a\cdot a(b+c-a)+b\cdot b(c+a-b)+c\cdot c(a+b-c)$$
$$\le a\cdot b(c+a-b)+b\cdot c(a+b-c)+c\cdot a(b+c-a) \qquad (2)$$

(1) + (2):
$2[a^2(b+c-a)+b^2(c+a-b)+c^2(a+b-c)]\le 6abc$
or $a^2(b+c-a)+b^2(c+a-b)+c^2(a+b-c)\le 3abc$

Example 11. Let a, b, c be non-negative real numbers. Prove that $\frac{a^3}{c^2+ac+a^2}+\frac{b^3}{a^2+ab+b^2}+\frac{c^3}{b^2+bc+c^2}\ge\frac{a+b+c}{3}$.

Solution:
Since the inequality is cyclic, we may assume without loss of generality that $a\le b\le c$ (or $a\le c\le b$).

We know that $a^2+ab+b^2\le c^2+ac+a^2 \le b^2+bc+c^2$.

We have the following two similarly ordered sequences:

a^3, b^3, c^3

$\frac{1}{b^2+bc+c^2}, \frac{1}{c^2+ac+a^2}, \frac{1}{a^2+ab+b^2}$.

By rearrangement inequality, we have

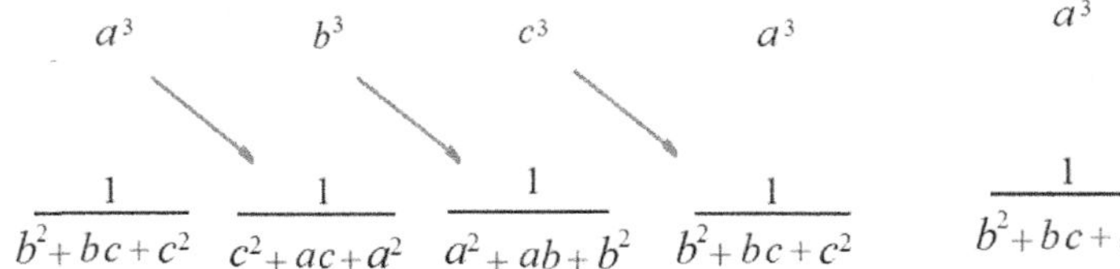

a^3 b^3 c^3

$\frac{1}{b^2+bc+c^2}$ $\frac{1}{c^2+ac+a^2}$ $\frac{1}{a^2+ab+b^2}$

$$\frac{a^3}{c^2+ac+a^2}+\frac{b^3}{a^2+ab+b^2}+\frac{c^3}{b^2+bc+c^2}\geq\frac{a^3}{a^2+ab+b^2}+\frac{b^3}{b^2+bc+c^2}+\frac{c^3}{c^2+ac+a^2} \quad (1)$$

We see that $\frac{a^3}{a^2+ab+b^2}=\frac{a^3+a^2b+ab^2-(a^2b+ab^2)}{a^2+ab+b^2}=a-\frac{a^2b+ab^2}{a^2+ab+b^2}=a-\frac{ab(a+b)}{a^2+ab+b^2}$

Note that $a^2+ab+b^2\leq 3ab$

$$\frac{a^3}{a^2+ab+b^2}=a-\frac{ab(a+b)}{a^2+ab+b^2}\geq a-\frac{ab(a+b)}{3ab}=a-\frac{a+b}{3}.$$

Similarly, $\frac{b^3}{b^2+bc+c^2}\geq b-\frac{b+c}{3}, \frac{c^3}{c^2+ac+a^2}\geq c-\frac{c+a}{3}$.

Substituting these values into (1):

$$\frac{a^3}{c^2+ac+a^2}+\frac{b^3}{a^2+ab+b^2}+\frac{c^3}{b^2+bc+c^2}\geq a-\frac{a+b}{3}+b-\frac{b+c}{3}+c-\frac{c+a}{3}$$

$$=a+b+c-\frac{2(a+b+c)}{3}$$

$$=\frac{a+b+c}{3}.$$

We can prove the case when $a\leq c\leq b$ similarly.

Example 12. Let a, b, c be non-negative real numbers. Prove that $\frac{a^3}{b^2+bc+c^2}+\frac{b^3}{c^2+ac+a^2}+\frac{c^3}{a^2+ab+b^2}\geq\frac{a^2+b^2+c^2}{a+b+c}$.

Solution:

Since the inequality is symmetrical, we may assume without loss of generality that $a \leq b \leq c$.

We know that $a^2+ab+b^2 \leq c^2+ac+a^2 \leq b^2+bc+c^2$.

We have the following two similarly ordered sequences:

a^3, b^3, c^3

$\frac{1}{b^2+bc+c^2}, \frac{1}{c^2+ac+a^2}, \frac{1}{a^2+ab+b^2}$.

By rearrangement inequality, we have

$$\begin{array}{ccc} a^3 & b^3 & c^3 \\ \downarrow & \downarrow & \downarrow \\ \frac{1}{b^2+bc+c^2} & \frac{1}{c^2+ac+a^2} & \frac{1}{a^2+ab+b^2} \end{array} \qquad \begin{array}{cccc} a^3 & b^3 & c^3 & a^3 \\ \nearrow & \nearrow & \nearrow & \\ \frac{1}{b^2+bc+c^2} & \frac{1}{c^2+ac+a^2} & \frac{1}{a^2+ab+b^2} & \frac{1}{b^2+bc+c^2} \end{array}$$

$$\begin{bmatrix} a^3 & b^3 & c^3 \\ \frac{1}{b^2+bc+c^2} & \frac{1}{c^2+ac+a^2} & \frac{1}{a^2+ab+b^2} \end{bmatrix} \geq \begin{bmatrix} a^3 & b^3 & c^3 \\ \frac{1}{a^2+ab+b^2} & \frac{1}{b^2+bc+c^2} & \frac{1}{c^2+ac+a^2} \end{bmatrix}$$

$$\frac{a^3}{b^2+bc+c^2}+\frac{b^3}{c^2+ac+a^2}+\frac{c^3}{a^2+ab+b^2}\geq\frac{a^3}{a^2+ab+b^2}+\frac{b^3}{b^2+bc+c^2}+\frac{c^3}{c^2+ac+a^2} \quad (1)$$

We know that

$$\frac{a^3}{a^2+ab+b^2}+\frac{b^3}{b^2+bc+c^2}+\frac{c^3}{c^2+ac+a^2}=\frac{a^4}{a(a^2+ab+b^2)}+\frac{b^4}{b(b^2+bc+c^2)}+\frac{c^4}{c(c^2+ac+a^2)}$$

By Cauchy, we have

$$\frac{a^4}{a(a^2+ab+b^2)}+\frac{b^4}{b(b^2+bc+c^2)}+\frac{c^4}{c(c^2+ac+a^2)}$$
$$\geq \frac{(a^2+b^2+c^2)^2}{a(a^2+ab+b^2)+b(b^2+bc+c^2)+c(c^2+ac+a^2)}$$

So it suffices to prove
$(a+b+c)(a^2+b^2+c^2) \geq a(a^2+ab+b^2)+b(b^2+bc+c^2)+c(c^2+ac+a^2)$

which is true.

Therefore,
or $\frac{a^3}{b^2+bc+c^2}+\frac{b^3}{c^2+ac+a^2}+\frac{c^3}{a^2+ab+b^2} \geq \frac{(a^2+b^2+c^2)^2}{(a+b)c)(a^2+b^2+c^2)}=\frac{a^2+b^2+c^2}{a+b+c}$.

Example 13. Let *a, b, c* be non-negative real numbers. Prove that $\frac{a^3}{b^2+bc+c^2}+\frac{b^3}{c^2+ac+a^2}+\frac{c^3}{a^2+ab+b^2} \geq \frac{a^3+b^3+c^3}{a^2+b^2+c^2}$.

Solution:

$$\frac{a^3}{b^2+bc+c^2}+\frac{b^3}{c^2+ac+a^2}+\frac{c^3}{a^2+ab+b^2}=\frac{a^6}{a^3(b^2+bc+c^2)}+\frac{b^6}{b^3(c^2+ac+a^2)}+\frac{c^6}{c^3(a^2+ab+b^2)}$$

By Cauchy, we have

$$\frac{a^6}{a^3(b^2+bc+c^2)}+\frac{b^6}{b^3(c^2+ac+a^2)}+\frac{c^6}{c^3(a^2+ab+b^2)}$$

$$\geq \frac{(a^3+b^3+c^3)^2}{a^3(b^2+bc+c^2)+b^3(c^2+ac+a^2)+c^3(a^2+ab+b^2)}$$

So it suffices to prove

$A=(a^2+b^2+c^2)(a^3+b^3+c^3)$

$\geq a^3(a^2+ab+b^2)+b^3(b^2+bc+c^2)+c^3(c^2+ac+a^2)=B$

$$A = a^5 + b^5 + c^5 + a^3b^2 + a^2b^3 + b^3c^2 + b^2c^3 + c^3a^2 + c^2a^3$$

$$B = a^3b^2 + a^3bc + a^3c^2 + b^3c^2 + b^3ca + b^3a^2 + c^3a^2 + c^3ab + c^3b^2$$

It suffices to prove

$$a^5 + b^5 + c^5 \geq a^3bc + b^3ca + c^3ab \qquad (1)$$

Since the above inequality is symmetrical, we may assume without loss of generality that $a \leq b \leq c$.

We have the following two similarly ordered sequences:

a, b, c
a, b, c
a, b, c
a, b, c
a, b, c

By rearrangement inequality, we have

$$\begin{bmatrix} a & b & c \\ a & b & c \\ a & b & c \\ a & b & c \\ a & b & c \end{bmatrix} \geq \begin{bmatrix} a & b & c \\ a & b & c \\ a & b & c \\ b & c & a \\ c & a & b \end{bmatrix}$$

$a^5 + b^5 + c^5 \geq a^3bc + b^3ca + c^3ab$

Therefore,

$$\frac{a^3}{b^2+bc+c^2} + \frac{b^3}{c^2+ac+a^2} + \frac{c^3}{a^2+ab+b^2}$$

$$\geq \frac{(a^3+b^3+c^3)^2}{a^3(b^2+bc+c^2)+b^3(c^2+ac+a^2)+c^3(a^2+ab+b^2)}$$

$$\geq \frac{(a^3+b^3+c^3)^2}{(a^2+b^2+c^2)(a^3+b^3+c^3)} = \frac{a^3+b^3+c^3}{a^2+b^2+c^2}.$$

Example 14. Let a, b, $c > 0$ such that $a + b + c = 1$. Prove that $\frac{a^2}{b} + \frac{b^2}{c} + \frac{c^2}{a} \geq 3(a^2 + b^2 + c^2)$.

Solution:

$$\frac{a^2}{b} + \frac{b^2}{c} + \frac{c^2}{a} = \frac{a^4}{a^2b} + \frac{b^4}{b^2c} + \frac{c^4}{c^2a}.$$

By Cauchy, $\frac{a^4}{a^2b} + \frac{b^4}{b^2c} + \frac{c^4}{c^2a} \geq \frac{(a^2+b^2+c^2)^2}{a^2b+b^2c+c^2a}$.

It remains to prove $\frac{(a^2+b^2+c^2)^2}{a^2b+b^2c+c^2a} \geq 3(a^2 + b^2 + c^2) \quad \Leftrightarrow$

$(a^2 + b^2 + c^2)(a + b + c) \geq 3(a^2b + b^2c + c^2a) \quad \Leftrightarrow$

$a^3 + b^3 + c^3 + ab^2 + bc^2 + ca^2 \geq 2(a^2b + b^2c + c^2a)$ (1)

We have the following similarly ordered sequences,

$a,\ b,\ c$

$a^2, b^2\ c^2$

By the rearrangement inequality, we have

$a \to a^2$, $b \to b^2$, $c \to c^2$ $\qquad$ $a^2 \nearrow b$, $b^2 \nearrow c$, $c^2 \nearrow a$

$a^3 + b^3 + c^3 \geq a^2b + b^2c + c^2a$ (2)

By the rearrangement inequality, we also have

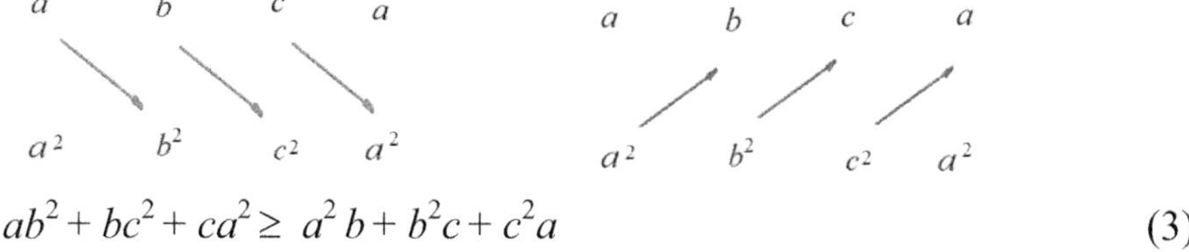

$ab^2 + bc^2 + ca^2 \geq a^2b + b^2c + c^2a$ (3)

Adding (2) and (3) we proved (1). QED.

Example 15. (1997 USA Math Olympiad) Prove that, for all positive real numbers a, b, c, $\frac{1}{a^3+b^3+abc}+\frac{1}{b^3+c^3+abc}+\frac{1}{c^3+a^3+abc} \le \frac{1}{abc}$.

Solution:
Method 1:
The given inequality can be written as

$$\frac{abc}{a^3+b^3+abc}+\frac{abc}{b^3+c^3+abc}+\frac{abc}{c^3+a^3+abc} \le 1$$

We know that the following two similarly ordered sequences:
a, b
a^2, b^2

By the rearrangement inequality, we have

$a \quad b \qquad\qquad a \quad b \quad a$

$\downarrow \quad \downarrow \qquad\qquad \searrow \quad \searrow$

$a^2 \quad b^2 \qquad\qquad a^2 \quad b^2 \quad a^2$

$a^3 + b^3 \ge a^2b + ab^2$.

Thus

$$\frac{abc}{a^3+b^3+abc} \le \frac{abc}{a^2b+ab^2+abc} \le \frac{abc}{ab(a+b+c)} = \frac{c}{a+b+c} \qquad (1)$$

Similarly

$$\frac{abc}{b^3+c^3+abc} \le \frac{a}{a+b+c} \qquad (2)$$

and

$$\frac{abc}{c^3+a^3+abc} \le \frac{b}{a+b+c} \qquad (3)$$

(1) + (2) + (3):

$$\frac{abc}{a^3+b^3+abc}+\frac{abc}{b^3+c^3+abc}+\frac{abc}{c^3+a^3+abc} \le 1 \text{, or}$$

$$\frac{1}{a^3+b^3+abc}+\frac{1}{b^3+c^3+abc}+\frac{1}{c^3+a^3+abc}\leq\frac{1}{abc}.$$

Method 2:

The inequality $(a-b)(a^2-b^2)\geq 0$ implies $a^3+b^3\geq ab(a+b)$, so

$$\frac{1}{a^3+b^3+abc}\leq\frac{1}{ab(a+b)+abc}=\frac{c}{abc(a+b+c)} \qquad (1)$$

Similarly

$$\frac{1}{b^3+c^3+abc}\leq\frac{1}{bc(b+c)+abc}=\frac{a}{abc(a+b+c)} \qquad (2)$$

and

$$\frac{1}{c^3+a^3+abc}\leq\frac{1}{ca(c+a)+abc}=\frac{b}{abc(a+b+c)} \qquad (3)$$

(1) + (2) + (3):

$$\frac{1}{a^3+b^3+abc}+\frac{1}{b^3+c^3+abc}+\frac{1}{c^3+a^3+abc}\leq\frac{a+b+c}{abc(a+b+c)}=\frac{1}{abc}.$$

CHAPTER 7. PROBLMES

Problem 1. (1996 Hungary Math Olympiad) Show that for real positive numbers $a, b,\ a+b=1,\ \frac{a^2}{a+1}+\frac{b^2}{b+1}\geq\frac{1}{3}$.

Problem 2. a, b, and c are positive real numbers. Show that

$$\frac{a^8+b^8+c^8}{a^2b^2c^2}\geq ab+bc+ca.$$

Problem 3. (1987 China IMO Team Training Problem) Prove that for all positive real numbers a, b, and c, $a^5+b^5+c^5\geq a^3bc+ab^3c+abc^3$.

Problem 4. (1974 USAMO) If $a, b, c > 0$, then prove that $a^a\, b^b\, c^c \geq (abc)^{(a+b+c)/3}$.

Problem 5. (2005 Germany Math Olympiad) If $a, b, c > 0$ and $a + b + c = 1$, show that $2(\frac{a}{b}+\frac{b}{c}+\frac{c}{a})\geq\frac{1+a}{1-a}+\frac{1+b}{1-b}+\frac{1+c}{1-c}$.

Problem 6. (United Kingdom, 1999) Three non-negative real numbers a, b and c satisfy $a + b + c = 1$. Prove that $7(ab + bc + ca) \leq 2 + 9abc$.

Problem 7. (2005 Austria) Show that for positive real numbers a, b, c, d, $\frac{1}{a^3}+\frac{1}{b^3}+\frac{1}{c^3}+\frac{1}{d^3}\geq\frac{a+b+c+d}{abcd}$.

Problem 8. (1962-1963 Poland Math Olympiad) Show that if a, b, c are positive real numbers, $a+b+c\leq\frac{a^4+b^4+c^4}{abc}$.

Problem 9. Let x, y, z be non-negative real numbers. Prove that $(x+y-z)(y+z-x)(z+x-y)\leq xyz$.

Problem 10. Let a, b, c be non-negative real numbers. Prove that $\frac{a^3}{b^2+bc+c^2}+\frac{b^3}{c^2+ac+a^2}+\frac{c^3}{a^2+ab+b^2}\geq\frac{a+b+c}{3}$.

Problem 11. Let a, b, c be non-negative real numbers. Prove that $\frac{a^2}{c^2+ac+a^2}+\frac{b^2}{a^2+ab+b^2}+\frac{c^2}{b^2+bc+c^2}\geq 1$.

Problem 12. (1997 Romania) Let x, y, z be non-negative real numbers with $xyz = 1$. Prove that $\frac{x^9+y^9}{x^6+x^3y^3+y^6}+\frac{y^9+z^9}{y^6+y^3z^3+z^6}+\frac{z^9+x^9}{z^6+z^3x^3+x^6}\geq 2$

Problem 13. (2007APMO) Let x, y, z be positive real numbers such that $\sqrt{x}+\sqrt{y}+\sqrt{z}=1$. Prove that $\frac{x^2+yz}{\sqrt{2x^2(y+z)}}+\frac{y^2+zx}{\sqrt{2y^2(z+x)}}+\frac{z^2+xy}{\sqrt{2z^2(x+y)}}\geq 1$.

Problem 14. (1996 IMO Short List**)** Prove that, for all positive real numbers a, b, c, and $abc = 1$, $\frac{ab}{a^5+b^5+ab}+\frac{bc}{b^5+c^5+bc}+\frac{ca}{c^5+a^5+ca}\leq 1$.

Problem 15. (1961 IMO) Let a, b, c be the lengths of a triangle whose area is S. Prove that $a^2+c^2+b^2\geq 4S\sqrt{3}$. In what case does equality hold?

CHAPTER 7. SOLUTIONS

Problem 1. Solution:

Since the inequality is symmetric, WLOG, we may assume that $a \le b$. Then we know that $a^2 \le b^2$.

Then we have the following two similarly ordered sequences:

a^2, b^2

$\frac{1}{b+1}, \frac{1}{a+1}$

Examine the rearrangement inequality, we see that $\frac{a^2}{a+1}$ and $\frac{b^2}{b+1}$ are oppositely sorted. So $\frac{a^2}{a+1} + \frac{b^2}{b+1}$ is the smallest term. Thus we are not able to use the rearrangement inequality to solve the problem.

$$\begin{matrix} a^2 & & b^2 \\ & \times & \\ \frac{1}{b+1} & & \frac{1}{a+1} \end{matrix}$$

We use the condition $a+b=1$ to rewrite the given inequality:

$$\frac{a^2}{(a+b)(a+a+b)} + \frac{b^2}{(a+b)(b+a+b)} \ge \frac{1}{3}$$

$$\Leftrightarrow \frac{a^2}{(a+b)(2a+b)} + \frac{b^2}{(a+b)(2b+a)} \ge \frac{1}{3} \qquad \Leftrightarrow \frac{a^2(2b+a)+b^2(2a+b)}{(a+b)(2a+b)(2b+a)} \ge \frac{1}{3}$$

$$\Leftrightarrow \quad \frac{a^3+b^3+2a^2b+2ab^2}{2a^3+2b^3+8a^2b+8ab^2} \ge \frac{1}{3}$$

$$\Leftrightarrow \quad 3(a^3+b^3+2a^2b+2ab^2) \ge 2a^3+2b^3+7a^2b+7ab^2$$

Which is equivalent to prove $a^3+b^3 \ge a^2b+ab^2$.

We know that the following two similarly ordered sequences:

a, b

a^2, b^2

By the rearrangement inequality, we have

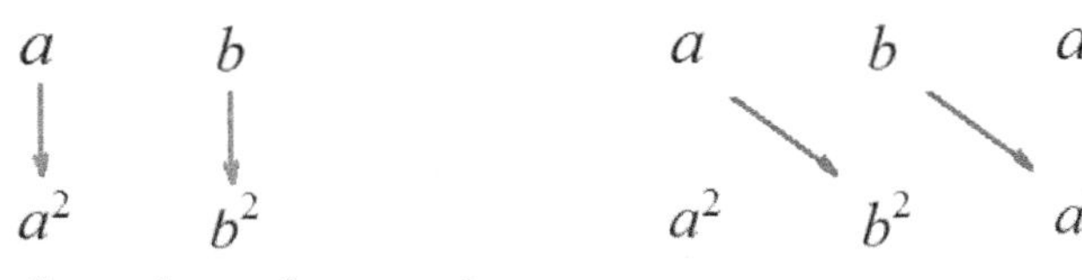

$a^3 + b^3 \geq a^2b + ab^2$.

The equality holds when $a = b = \frac{1}{3}$.

Method 2:

By Cauchy, $\frac{a^2}{a+1} + \frac{b^2}{b+1} \geq \frac{(a+b)^2}{a+1+b+1} = \frac{1}{3}$.

Problem 2. Solution:

$\frac{a^8+b^8+c^8}{a^2b^2c^2} \geq ab + bc + ca \Leftrightarrow a^8 + b^8 + c^8 \geq a^2b^3c^3 + a^3b^2c^3 + a^2b^3c^2$.

Since the inequality is symmetric, WLOG, we may assume that $a \leq b \leq c$. Then we know that $a^2 \leq b^2 \leq c^2$, a^3, b^3, c^3.

Then we have the following three similarly ordered sequences:

a^2, b^2, c^2.

a^3, b^3, c^3.

a^3, b^3, c^3.

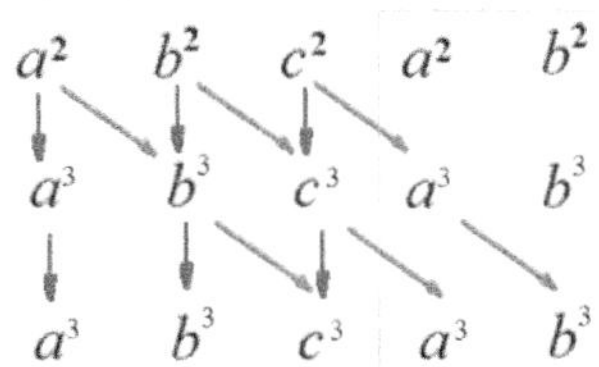

By the rearrangement inequality, we have $a^8 + b^8 + c^8 \geq a^2b^3c^3 + a^3b^2c^3 + a^2b^3c^2$.

Problem 3. Proof:

The given inequality can be written as

$\frac{a^4}{bc} + \frac{b^4}{ca} + \frac{c^4}{ab} \geq a^2 + b^2 + c^2$.

Since the inequality is symmetric, WLOG, we may assume that $a \le b \le c$. Then we know that $a^4 \le b^4 \le c^4$.

Then we have the following two similarly ordered sequences:

a^4, b^4, c^4.

$\frac{1}{bc}, \frac{1}{ac}, \frac{1}{ab}$

By the rearrangement inequality, we have

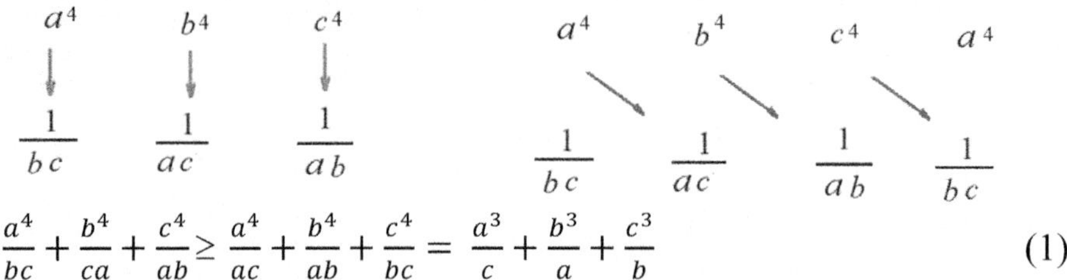

$$\frac{a^4}{bc} + \frac{b^4}{ca} + \frac{c^4}{ab} \ge \frac{a^4}{ac} + \frac{b^4}{ab} + \frac{c^4}{bc} = \frac{a^3}{c} + \frac{b^3}{a} + \frac{c^3}{b} \qquad (1)$$

Then we have the following two similarly ordered sequences:

a^3, b^3, c^3.

$\frac{1}{c}, \frac{1}{b}, \frac{1}{a}$

By the rearrangement inequality, we have

$$\frac{a^3}{c} + \frac{b^3}{a} + \frac{c^3}{b} \ge \frac{a^3}{a} + \frac{c^3}{c} + \frac{b^3}{b} = a^2 + b^2 + c^2 .$$

Problem 4. Solution:

By symmetry we may assume $a \le b \le c$, then $\ln a \le \ln b \le \ln c$.

For the following similarly ordered two sequences,

a, b, c,

$\ln a$, $\ln b$, $\ln c$

by the rearrangement inequality, we have

$$\begin{array}{ccc} a & b & c \\ \downarrow & \downarrow & \downarrow \\ \ln a & \ln b & \ln c \end{array} \qquad \begin{array}{cccc} a & b & c & a \\ \searrow & \searrow & \searrow & \\ \ln a & \ln b & \ln c & \ln a \end{array} \qquad \begin{array}{cccc} a & b & c & a \\ \nearrow & \nearrow & \nearrow & \\ \ln a & \ln b & \ln c & \ln a \end{array}$$

$a\ln a + b\ln b + c\ln c \geq c\ln a + a\ln b + b\ln c$ (1)

$a\ln a + b\ln b + c\ln c \geq b\ln a + c\ln b + a\ln c$ (2)

$a\ln a + b\ln b + c\ln c \geq a\ln a + b\ln b + c\ln c$ (3)

(1) + (2) + (3):

$3(a\ln a + b\ln b + c\ln c) \geq (a + b + c)(\ln a + \ln b + \ln c) \quad \Rightarrow$

$a\ln a + b\ln b + c\ln c \geq \frac{1}{3}(a + b + c)[\ln(abc)] \quad \Rightarrow$

$\ln(a^a b^b c^c) \geq \ln(abc)^{\frac{1}{3}(a+b+c)} \quad \Rightarrow \quad (a^a b^b c^c) \geq (abc)^{\frac{1}{3}(a+b+c)}$.

Problem 5. Solution:

The given inequality can be written as $\frac{a}{b} + \frac{b}{c} + \frac{c}{a} \geq \frac{3}{2} + \frac{a}{b+c} + \frac{b}{c+a} + \frac{c}{a+b}$,

Or $\frac{ab}{c(b+c)} + \frac{bc}{a(c+a)} + \frac{ca}{b(a+b)} \geq \frac{3}{2}$.

By the symmetrical property, we assume that $a \leq b \leq c$.

Then we have $\frac{1}{b+c} \leq \frac{1}{a+c} \leq \frac{1}{a+b}$, and

$\frac{ab}{c} \leq \frac{ca}{b} \leq \frac{bc}{a}$

For the following similarly ordered sequences,

$\frac{ab}{c}, \frac{ca}{b}, \frac{bc}{a}$

$\frac{1}{b+c}, \frac{1}{a+c}, \frac{1}{a+b}$,

based on the rearrangement inequality,

$\frac{ab}{c}$ $\frac{ca}{b}$ $\frac{bc}{a}$ $\frac{ab}{c}$ $\frac{ca}{b}$ $\frac{bc}{a}$

$\frac{1}{(b+c)}$ $\frac{1}{(c+a)}$ $\frac{1}{(a+b)}$ $\frac{1}{(b+c)}$ $\frac{1}{(c+a)}$ $\frac{1}{(a+b)}$

$$\frac{ab}{c(b+c)}+\frac{bc}{a(c+a)}+\frac{ca}{b(a+b)} \geq \frac{ab}{c(a+b)}+\frac{bc}{a(b+c)}+\frac{ca}{b(c+a)}.$$

Let $ab = x$, $bc = y$, and $ca = z$.

$\frac{ab}{c(a+b)}+\frac{bc}{a(b+c)}+\frac{ca}{b(c+a)}$ can be written as $\frac{ab}{c(a+b)}+\frac{bc}{a(b+c)}+\frac{ca}{b(c+a)} = \frac{x}{z+y)}+\frac{y}{x+z}+\frac{z}{y+x}$, which is the Nesbitt's Inequality and we know that $\frac{x}{z+y)}+\frac{y}{x+z}+\frac{z}{y+x} \geq \frac{3}{2}$. QED.

Problem 6. Solution.

The given inequality can be written as the following inequalities:

$7(ab+bc+ca) \leq 2+9abc$

$\Leftrightarrow 7(ab+bc+ca)(a+b+c) \leq 2(a+b+c)^3+9abc$

$\Leftrightarrow a^2b+a\,b^2+b^2c+b\,c^2+c^2a+c\,a^2 \leq 2(a^3+b^3+c^3)$ (1)

For the following similarly ordered sequences,

$a,\ b,\ c$

$a^2, b^2\ c^2$

By the rearrangement inequality, we have

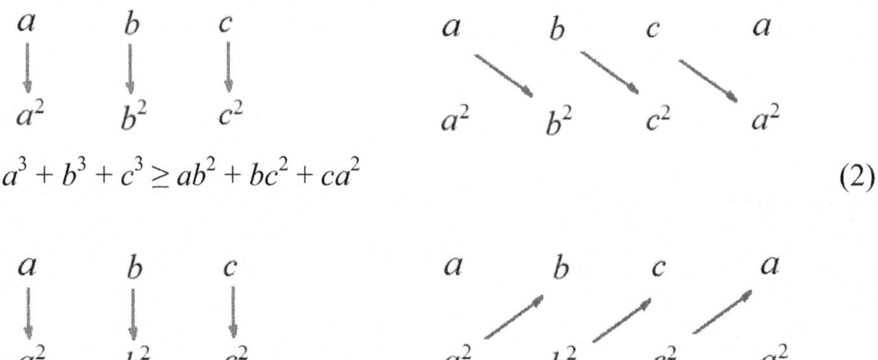

$a^3+b^3+c^3 \geq ab^2+bc^2+ca^2$ (2)

$$a^3 + b^3 + c^3 \geq a^2b + b^2c + c^2a \qquad (3)$$

(2) + (3):
$$2(a^3 + b^3 + c^3) \geq ab^2 + bc^2 + ca^2 + a^2b + b^2c + c^2a.$$

Problem 7. Solution:
The given inequality is equivalent to the following inequality:
$$\frac{1}{a^3} + \frac{1}{b^3} + \frac{1}{c^3} + \frac{1}{d^3} \geq \frac{1}{abc} + \frac{1}{abd} + \frac{1}{acd} + \frac{1}{bcd}.$$

Since the expression is a symmetric function of a, b, c, and d, we can assume, without loss of generality, that $a \leq b \leq c \leq d$, and $\frac{1}{d} \leq \frac{1}{c} \leq \frac{1}{b} \leq \frac{1}{a}$.

Then we have the following two similarly ordered sequences:
$$\frac{1}{d}, \frac{1}{c}, \frac{1}{b}, \frac{1}{a}$$
$$\frac{1}{d}, \frac{1}{c}, \frac{1}{b}, \frac{1}{a}$$
$$\frac{1}{d}, \frac{1}{c}, \frac{1}{b}, \frac{1}{a}$$

By the rearrangement inequality,

$$\begin{array}{cccc} \frac{1}{d} & \frac{1}{c} & \frac{1}{b} & \frac{1}{a} \\ \downarrow & \downarrow & \downarrow & \downarrow \\ \frac{1}{d} & \frac{1}{c} & \frac{1}{b} & \frac{1}{a} \\ \downarrow & \downarrow & \downarrow & \downarrow \\ \frac{1}{d} & \frac{1}{c} & \frac{1}{b} & \frac{1}{a} \end{array} \qquad \begin{array}{cccccc} \frac{1}{d} & \frac{1}{c} & \frac{1}{b} & \frac{1}{a} & \frac{1}{d} & \frac{1}{c} \\ \frac{1}{d} & \frac{1}{c} & \frac{1}{b} & \frac{1}{a} & \frac{1}{d} & \frac{1}{c} \\ \frac{1}{d} & \frac{1}{c} & \frac{1}{b} & \frac{1}{a} & \frac{1}{d} & \frac{1}{c} \end{array}$$

$$\frac{1}{a^3} + \frac{1}{b^3} + \frac{1}{c^3} + \frac{1}{d^3} \geq \frac{1}{dcb} + \frac{1}{cba} + \frac{1}{bad} + \frac{1}{adc}.$$

Problem 8. Proof:
$$a^{n+1} + b^{n+1} + c^{n+1} \geq (a^{n-2} + b^{n-2} + c^{n-2})abc.$$

Let $n = 3$, $a^{3+1} + b^{3+1} + c^{3+1} \geq (a^{3-2} + b^{3-2} + c^{3-2})abc = (a + b + c)abc$.

Dividing both sides by abc: $\quad a + b + c \leq \frac{a^4+b^4+c^4}{abc}$.

Problem 9. Solution:

Let $x = a + b$, $y = b + c$, and $z = c + a$.

The given inequality can be written as

$(a + b + b + c - c - a)(b + c + c + a - a - b)(c + a + a + b - b - c) \leq (a + b)(b + c)(c + a)$.

Or $(a + b)(b + c)(c + a) \geq 8abc$ (1)

We have the following two similarly ordered sequences:

$\sqrt{a}$, $\sqrt{b}$

$\sqrt{a}$, $\sqrt{b}$

By the rearrangement inequality, we have

$\sqrt{a}$ $\sqrt{b}$ $\sqrt{a}$ $\sqrt{b}$

$\sqrt{a}$ $\sqrt{b}$ $\sqrt{a}$ $\sqrt{b}$

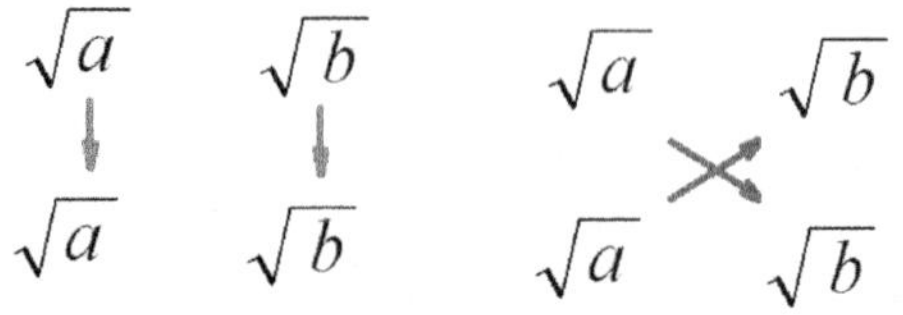

$\sqrt{a} \cdot \sqrt{a} + \sqrt{b} \cdot \sqrt{b} = a + b \geq \sqrt{a} \cdot \sqrt{b} + \sqrt{a} \cdot \sqrt{b} = 2\sqrt{ab}$ (1)

We can have the following two similarly ordered sequences:

$\sqrt{b}$, $\sqrt{c}$

$\sqrt{b}$, $\sqrt{c}$

By the rearrangement inequality, we have

$\sqrt{b}$ $\sqrt{c}$ $\sqrt{b}$ $\sqrt{c}$

$\sqrt{b}$ $\sqrt{c}$ $\sqrt{b}$ $\sqrt{c}$

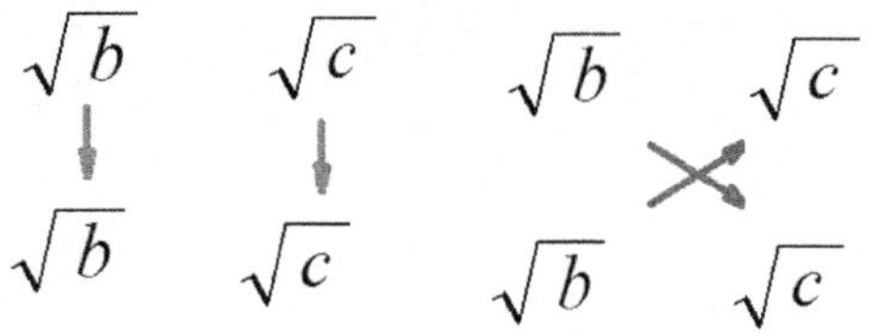

$\sqrt{b} \cdot \sqrt{b} + \sqrt{c} \cdot \sqrt{c} = b + c \geq \sqrt{b} \cdot \sqrt{b} + \sqrt{c} \cdot \sqrt{c} = 2\sqrt{bc}$ (2)

We can have the following two similarly ordered sequences:

$\sqrt{c}$, $\sqrt{a}$

$\sqrt{c}$, $\sqrt{a}$

By the rearrangement inequality, we have

$$\begin{matrix} \sqrt{c} & \sqrt{a} \\ \downarrow & \downarrow \\ \sqrt{c} & \sqrt{a} \end{matrix} \qquad \begin{matrix} \sqrt{c} & & \sqrt{a} \\ & \times & \\ \sqrt{c} & & \sqrt{a} \end{matrix}$$

$$\sqrt{c}\cdot\sqrt{c}+\sqrt{a}\cdot\sqrt{a}=c+a\geq\sqrt{c}\cdot\sqrt{a}+\sqrt{c}\cdot\sqrt{a}=2\sqrt{ca} \qquad (3)$$

$(1)\times(2)\times(3)$:

$$(a+b)(b+c)(c+a)\geq(2\sqrt{ab})(2\sqrt{bc})(2\sqrt{ca})=8abc$$

The proof is finished. Equality holds for $x=y=z$ and $x=y$, $z=0$ and permutations.

Problem 10. Solution:

Method 1:

Since the inequality is symmetrical, we may assume without loss of generality that $a\leq b\leq c$.

We know that $a^2+ab+b^2\leq c^2+ac+a^2\leq b^2+bc+c^2$.

We have the following two similarly ordered sequences:

a^3, b^3, c^3

$\frac{1}{b^2+bc+c^2}, \frac{1}{c^2+ac+a^2}, \frac{1}{a^2+ab+b^2}$.

By rearrangement inequality, we have

$$\begin{matrix} a^3 & b^3 & c^3 \\ \downarrow & \downarrow & \downarrow \\ \frac{1}{b^2+bc+c^2} & \frac{1}{c^2+ac+a^2} & \frac{1}{a^2+ab+b^2} \end{matrix} \qquad \begin{matrix} a^3 & & b^3 & & c^3 & & a^3 \\ & \searrow & & \searrow & & \searrow & \\ \frac{1}{b^2+bc+c^2} & & \frac{1}{c^2+ac+a^2} & & \frac{1}{a^2+ab+b^2} & & \frac{1}{b^2+bc+c^2} \end{matrix}$$

Or $\begin{bmatrix} a^3 & b^3 & c^3 \\ \frac{1}{b^2+bc+c^2} & \frac{1}{c^2+ac+a^2} & \frac{1}{a^2+ab+b^2} \end{bmatrix} \geq \begin{bmatrix} a^3 & b^3 & c^3 \\ \frac{1}{c^2+ac+a^2} & \frac{1}{a^2+ab+b^2} & \frac{1}{b^2+bc+c^2} \end{bmatrix}$

$$\frac{a^3}{b^2+bc+c^2}+\frac{b^3}{c^2+ac+a^2}+\frac{c^3}{a^2+ab+b^2}\geq\frac{a^3}{c^2+ac+a^2}+\frac{b^3}{a^2+ab+b^2}+\frac{c^3}{b^2+bc+c^2} \qquad (1)$$

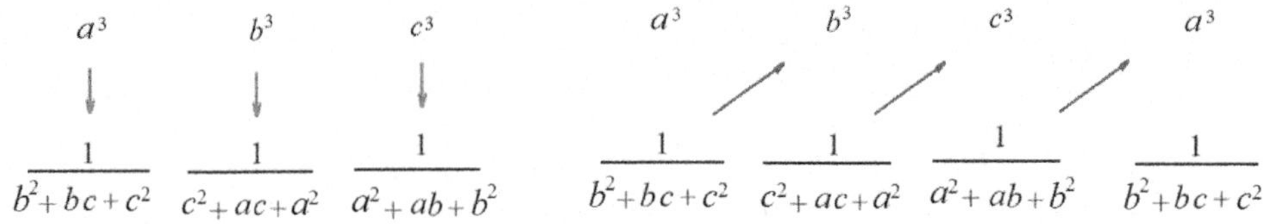

$$\begin{array}{ccc} a^3 & b^3 & c^3 \\ \downarrow & \downarrow & \downarrow \\ \frac{1}{b^2+bc+c^2} & \frac{1}{c^2+ac+a^2} & \frac{1}{a^2+ab+b^2} \end{array} \qquad \begin{array}{cccc} & a^3 & b^3 & c^3 \quad a^3 \\ & \nearrow & \nearrow & \nearrow \\ \frac{1}{b^2+bc+c^2} & \frac{1}{c^2+ac+a^2} & \frac{1}{a^2+ab+b^2} & \frac{1}{b^2+bc+c^2} \end{array}$$

$$\begin{bmatrix} a^3 & b^3 & c^3 \\ \frac{1}{b^2+bc+c^2} & \frac{1}{c^2+ac+a^2} & \frac{1}{a^2+ab+b^2} \end{bmatrix} \geq \begin{bmatrix} a^3 & b^3 & c^3 \\ \frac{1}{a^2+ab+b^2} & \frac{1}{b^2+bc+c^2} & \frac{1}{c^2+ac+a^2} \end{bmatrix}$$

$$\frac{a^3}{b^2+bc+c^2}+\frac{b^3}{c^2+ac+a^2}+\frac{c^3}{a^2+ab+b^2}\geq\frac{a^3}{a^2+ab+b^2}+\frac{b^3}{b^2+bc+c^2}+\frac{c^3}{c^2+ac+a^2} \qquad (2)$$

(1) + (2):

$$2\left(\frac{a^3}{b^2+bc+c^2}+\frac{b^3}{c^2+ac+a^2}+\frac{c^3}{a^2+ab+b^2}\right)\geq\frac{a^3+c^3}{c^2+ac+a^2}+\frac{b^3+a^3}{a^2+ab+b^2}+\frac{c^3+b^3}{b^2+bc+c^2}.$$

Note that $\frac{a^3+c^3}{c^2+ac+a^2}\geq\frac{a+c}{3}$, $\frac{b^3+a^3}{a^2+ab+b^2}\geq\frac{b+a}{3}$, $\frac{c^3+b^3}{b^2+bc+c^2}\geq\frac{c+b}{3}$, we get

$$2\left(\frac{a^3}{b^2+bc+c^2}+\frac{b^3}{c^2+ac+a^2}+\frac{c^3}{a^2+ab+b^2}\right)\geq\frac{a+c}{3}+\frac{b+a}{3}+\frac{c+b}{3}=\frac{2(a+b+c)}{3}.$$

or $\frac{a^3}{b^2+bc+c^2}+\frac{b^3}{c^2+ac+a^2}+\frac{c^3}{a^2+ab+b^2}\geq\frac{a+b+c}{3}$.

Method 2:

We know that $\frac{a^3}{b^2-bc+c^2}+\frac{b^3}{c^2-ac+a^2}+\frac{c^3}{a^2-ab+b^2}\geq a+b+c$.

We also have

$(a-b)^2\geq 0 \Leftrightarrow a^2-2ab+b^2\geq 0 \Leftrightarrow 2a^2-4ab+2b^2\geq 0$

$\Leftrightarrow \quad 3a^2-3ab+3b^2\geq a^2+ab+b^2 \Leftrightarrow 3(a^2-ab+b^2)\geq a^2+ab+b^2$.

Thus we have

$a^2+ab+b^2\leq 3(a^2-ab+b^2)$,

$b^2 + bc + c^2 \le 3(b^2 - bc + c^2)$,
$c^2 + ac + a^2 \le 3(c^2 - ac + a^2)$.

Therefore,

$$\frac{a^3}{b^2+bc+c^2} + \frac{b^3}{c^2+ac+a^2} + \frac{c^3}{a^2+ab+b^2} \ge \frac{1}{3}\left(\frac{a^3}{b^2-bc+c^2} + \frac{b^3}{c^2-ac+a^2} + \frac{c^3}{a^2-ab+b^2}\right) \ge \frac{a+b+c}{3}.$$

QED.

Problem 11. Solution:

Since the inequality is cyclic, we may assume without loss of generality that $a \le b \le c$ (or $a \le c \le b$).

We know that $a^2 + ab + b^2 \le c^2 + ac + a^2 \le b^2 + bc + c^2$.

We have the following two similarly ordered sequences:

a^2, b^2, c^2

$\frac{1}{b^2+bc+c^2}, \frac{1}{c^2+ac+a^2}, \frac{1}{a^2+ab+b^2}$.

By rearrangement inequality, we have

$a^2 \quad b^2 \quad c^2 \quad a^2$

$\frac{1}{b^2+bc+c^2} \quad \frac{1}{c^2+ac+a^2} \quad \frac{1}{a^2+ab+b^2} \quad \frac{1}{b^2+bc+c^2}$

$a^2 \quad b^2 \quad c^2$

$\frac{1}{b^2+bc+c^2} \quad \frac{1}{c^2+ac+a^2} \quad \frac{1}{a^2+ab+b^2}$

$$\frac{a^2}{c^2+ac+a^2} + \frac{b^2}{a^2+ab+b^2} + \frac{c^2}{b^2+bc+c^2} \ge \frac{a^2}{a^2+ab+b^2} + \frac{b^2}{b^2+bc+c^2} + \frac{c^2}{c^2+ac+a^2} \qquad (1)$$

We see that

$$\frac{a^2}{a^2+ab+b^2} = \frac{a^2+ab+b^2-(ab+b^2)}{a^2+ab+b^2} = 1 - \frac{b(a+b)}{a^2+ab+b^2} \ge 1 - \frac{ba}{a^2+ab+b^2} - \frac{b^2}{a^2+ab+b^2}$$

Similarly, $\frac{b^2}{b^2+bc+c^2} \ge 1 - \frac{bc}{b^2+bc+c^2} - \frac{c^2}{b^2+bc+c^2}$,

$\frac{c^2}{c^2+ac+a^2} \ge 1 - \frac{ca}{c^2+ac+a^2} - \frac{a^2}{c^2+ac+a^2}$.

The right-hand side of (1) then can be written as

$$\frac{a^2}{a^2+ab+b^2}+\frac{b^2}{b^2+bc+c^2}+\frac{c^2}{c^2+ac+a^2}\ge 3-\frac{ba}{a^2+ab+b^2}-\frac{b^2}{a^2+ab+b^2}-\frac{bc}{b^2+bc+c^2}-\frac{c^2}{b^2+bc+c^2}-\frac{ca}{c^2+ac+a^2}-\frac{a^2}{c^2+ac+a^2}.$$

Or

$$2\left(\frac{a^2}{a^2+ab+b^2}+\frac{b^2}{b^2+bc+c^2}+\frac{c^2}{c^2+ac+a^2}\right)\ge 3-\frac{ba}{a^2+ab+b^2}-\frac{bc}{b^2+bc+c^2}-\frac{ca}{c^2+ac+a^2}.$$

$$\ge 3-\frac{ba}{3ab}-\frac{bc}{3bc}-\frac{ca}{3ac}=2.$$

Thus $\frac{a^2}{a^2+ab+b^2}+\frac{b^2}{b^2+bc+c^2}+\frac{c^2}{c^2+ac+a^2}\ge 1$

That is,

$$\frac{a^3}{c^2+ac+a^2}+\frac{b^3}{a^2+ab+b^2}+\frac{c^3}{b^2+bc+c^2}\ge\frac{a^2}{a^2+ab+b^2}+\frac{b^2}{b^2+bc+c^2}+\frac{c^2}{c^2+ac+a^2}\ge 1.$$

We can prove the case when $a \le c \le b$ similarly.

Problem 12. Solution:

Let $a = x^3$, $b = y^3$, and $c = z^3$. We have $abc = 1$. The original inequality is equivalent to (1):

$$\frac{a^3+b^3}{a^2+ab+b^2}+\frac{b^3+c^3}{b^2+bc+c^2}+\frac{c^3+a^3}{c^2+ac+a^2}\ge 2 \qquad (1)$$

We know that the following two similarly ordered sequences:

a, b

a^2, b^2

By the rearrangement inequality, we have

$$\begin{matrix} a & b \\ \downarrow & \downarrow \\ a^2 & b^2 \end{matrix} \qquad \begin{matrix} a & & b & & a \\ & \searrow & & \searrow & \\ a^2 & & b^2 & & a^2 \end{matrix}$$

$a^3+b^3\ge a^2b+ab^2.$

$$\frac{a^3+b^3}{a^2+ab+b^2}=\frac{3(a^3+b^3)}{3(a^2+ab+b^2)}=\frac{a^3+b^3+2(a^3+b^3)}{3(a^2+ab+b^2)}$$

$$\geq \frac{a^3+b^3+2(a^2b+ab^2)}{3(a^2+ab+b^2)} = \frac{a^3+b^3+2ab(a+b)}{3(a^2+ab+b^2)}$$

$$= \frac{(a+b)(a^2-ab+b^2)+2ab(a+b)}{3(a^2+ab+b^2)}$$

$$= \frac{(a+b)(a^2-ab+b^2+2ab)}{3(a^2+ab+b^2)}$$
$$= \frac{(a+b)(a^2+ab+b^2)}{3(a^2+ab+b^2)}$$
$$= \frac{a+b}{3}$$

Similarly
$$\frac{b^3+c^3}{b^2+bc+c^2} \geq \frac{b+c}{3}$$
$$\frac{c^3+a^3}{c^2+ac+a^2} \geq \frac{c+a}{3}$$

Thus we have
$$\frac{a^3+b^3}{a^2+ab+b^2} + \frac{b^3+c^3}{b^2+bc+c^2} + \frac{c^3+a^3}{c^2+ac+a^2} \geq \frac{a+b}{3} + \frac{b+c}{3} + \frac{c+a}{3}$$

$$= \frac{2(a+b+c)}{3} \geq \frac{2\cdot 3\sqrt[3]{abc}}{3} = 2.$$

Problem 13. Solution:
Since the inequality is symmetrical, we may assume without loss of generality that $x \leq y \leq z$.

We know that $x+y \leq x+z \leq y+z$, $xy \leq xz \leq yz$, $2x^2(y+z) \leq 2x^2(z+x) \leq 2z^2(x+y)$, and $\frac{1}{\sqrt{2z^2(x+y)}} \leq \frac{1}{\sqrt{2y^2(z+x)}} \leq \frac{1}{\sqrt{2x^2(y+z)}}$.

We have the following two similarly ordered sequences:

xy, xz, yz

$\frac{1}{\sqrt{2z^2(x+y)}}, \frac{1}{\sqrt{2y^2(z+x)}}, \frac{1}{\sqrt{2x^2(y+z)}}$

By rearrangement inequality, we have

$$\begin{array}{ccc} xy & xz & yz \\ \downarrow & \downarrow & \downarrow \\ \frac{1}{\sqrt{2z^2(x+y)}} & \frac{1}{\sqrt{2y^2(z+x)}} & \frac{1}{\sqrt{2x^2(y+z)}} \end{array} \qquad \begin{array}{cccc} xy & xz & yz & xy \\ \searrow & \searrow & \searrow & \\ \frac{1}{\sqrt{2z^2(x+y)}} & \frac{1}{\sqrt{2y^2(z+x)}} & \frac{1}{\sqrt{2x^2(y+z)}} & \frac{1}{\sqrt{2z^2(x+y)}} \end{array}$$

$$\frac{xy}{\sqrt{2z^2(x+y)}} + \frac{zx}{\sqrt{2y^2(z+x)}} + \frac{yz}{\sqrt{2x^2(y+z)}} \geq \frac{yz}{\sqrt{2z^2(x+y)}} + \frac{xy}{\sqrt{2y^2(z+x)}} + \frac{xz}{\sqrt{2x^2(y+z)}} \qquad (1)$$

$$\begin{array}{ccc} xy & xz & yz \\ \downarrow & \downarrow & \downarrow \\ \frac{1}{\sqrt{2z^2(x+y)}} & \frac{1}{\sqrt{2y^2(z+x)}} & \frac{1}{\sqrt{2x^2(y+z)}} \end{array} \qquad \begin{array}{cccc} xy & xz & yz & xy \\ \nearrow & \nearrow & \nearrow & \\ \frac{1}{\sqrt{2z^2(x+y)}} & \frac{1}{\sqrt{2y^2(z+x)}} & \frac{1}{\sqrt{2x^2(y+z)}} & \frac{1}{\sqrt{2z^2(x+y)}} \end{array}$$

$$\frac{xy}{\sqrt{2z^2(x+y)}} + \frac{zx}{\sqrt{2y^2(z+x)}} + \frac{yz}{\sqrt{2x^2(y+z)}} \geq \frac{xz}{\sqrt{2z^2(x+y)}} + \frac{yz}{\sqrt{2y^2(z+x)}} + \frac{xy}{\sqrt{2x^2(y+z)}} \qquad (2)$$

(1) + (2):

$$\frac{2xy}{\sqrt{2z^2(x+y)}} + \frac{2zx}{\sqrt{2y^2(z+x)}} + \frac{2yz}{\sqrt{2x^2(y+z)}} \geq \frac{xz+yz}{\sqrt{2z^2(x+y)}} + \frac{yz+xy}{\sqrt{2y^2(z+x)}} + \frac{xy+xz}{\sqrt{2x^2(y+z)}} \qquad (3)$$

Adding $\frac{2x^2}{\sqrt{2x^2(y+z)}} + \frac{2y^2}{\sqrt{2y^2(z+x)}} + \frac{2z^2}{\sqrt{2z^2(x+y)}}$ to both sides of (3):

$$2\left(\frac{x^2+yz}{\sqrt{2x^2(y+z)}} + \frac{y^2+zx}{\sqrt{2y^2(z+x)}} + \frac{z^2+xy}{\sqrt{2z^2(x+y)}}\right) \geq \frac{2z^2+xz+yz}{\sqrt{2z^2(x+y)}} + \frac{2y^2+yz+xy}{\sqrt{2y^2(z+x)}} + \frac{2x^2+xy+xz}{\sqrt{2x^2(y+z)}}.$$

$$= \frac{2z^2+z(x+y)}{\sqrt{2z^2(x+y)}} + \frac{2y^2+y(z+x)}{\sqrt{2y^2(z+x)}} + \frac{2x^2+x(y+z)}{\sqrt{2x^2(y+z)}}$$

$$\geq \frac{2\sqrt{2z^2 \times z(x+y)}}{\sqrt{2z^2(x+y)}} + \frac{2\sqrt{2y^2 \times y(z+x)}}{\sqrt{2y^2(z+x)}} + \frac{\sqrt{2x^2 \times x(y+z)}}{\sqrt{2x^2(y+z)}}$$

$= 2\sqrt{z} + 2\sqrt{y} + 2\sqrt{x} = 2(\sqrt{z} + \sqrt{y} + \sqrt{x}) = 2.$

Thus we proved $\frac{x^2+yz}{\sqrt{2x^2(y+z)}} + \frac{y^2+zx}{\sqrt{2y^2(z+x)}} + \frac{z^2+xy}{\sqrt{2z^2(x+y)}} \geq 1.$

Problem 14. Solution:

Method 1:

We know that the following two similarly ordered sequences:

a, b

a^2, b^2

By the rearrangement inequality, we have

$$\begin{matrix} a^2 & b^2 \\ \downarrow & \downarrow \\ a^3 & b^3 \end{matrix} \qquad \begin{matrix} a^2 & & b^2 & & a^2 \\ & \nearrow & & \nearrow & \\ a^3 & & b^3 & & a^3 \end{matrix}$$

$a^5 + b^5 \geq a^3b^2 + b^3a^2.$

Thus

$$\frac{ab}{a^5+b^5+ab} \leq \frac{ab}{a^3b^2+b^3a^2+ab} = \frac{abc^2}{a^2b^2c^2(a+b)+abc^2}$$
$$= \frac{(abc)c}{(abc)^2(a+b)+(abc)c} = \frac{c}{a+b+c} \qquad (1)$$

Similarly

$$\frac{bc}{b^5+c^5+bc} \leq \frac{a}{a+b+c} \qquad (2)$$

and

$$\frac{ca}{c^5+a^5+ca} \leq \frac{b}{a+b+c} \qquad (3)$$

(1) + (2) + (3):

$$\frac{ab}{a^5+b^5+ab} + \frac{bc}{b^5+c^5+bc} + \frac{ca}{c^5+a^5+ca} \leq 1 .$$

Equality holds if and only if $a = b = c = 1$.

Problem 15. Solution:

We know that $S = \sqrt{s(s-a)(s-b)(s-c)}$, where $s = \frac{a+b+c}{2}$.

After we do the substitution, the original inequality is equivalent to
$a^4 + b^4 + c^4 \geq a^2b^2 + b^2c^2a + c^2a^2$.

Since the inequality is symmetric, WLOG, we may assume that
$a \leq b \leq c$ and $a^2 \leq b^2 \leq c^2$.

For the following two sequences,
$a^2, b^2\ c^2$
$a^2, b^2\ c^2$
by the rearrangement inequality, we have

$$\begin{array}{ccccccc} a^2 & b^2 & c^2 & a^2 & b^2 & c^2 & a^2 \\ \downarrow & \downarrow & \downarrow & & \searrow & \searrow & \searrow \\ a^2 & b^2 & c^2 & a^2 & b^2 & c^2 & a^2 \end{array}$$

$a^4 + b^4 + c^4 \geq a^2b^2 + b^2c^2a + c^2a^2$
The equality holds when $a = b = c$, or when the triangle is equilateral.

Chapter 8. Finding Greatest/Smallest Values

Example 1. If $a, b, c \geq 0$, $a + b + c = 1$, find the greatest value of $ab + bc + ca$.

Solution: $\frac{1}{3}$.
For the following similarly ordered sequences,
$a, \ b, \ c$
$a, \ b, \ c$

by the rearrangement inequality, we have

a b c   a b c a
a b c   a b c a

$a^2 + b^2 + c^2 \geq ab + bc + ca$, or
$ab + bc + ca \leq a^2 + b^2 + c^2 = (a + b + c)^2 - 2(ab + bc + ca)$, or

$3(ab + bc + ca) \leq (a + b + c)^2 = 1 \qquad \Rightarrow \qquad ab + bc + ca \leq \frac{1}{3}$.
The greatest value $\frac{1}{3}$ is achieved when $a = b = c = \frac{1}{3}$.

Example 2. If $a, b, c \geq 0$, $a + b + c = 1$, find the greatest value of $a\sqrt{b} + b\sqrt{c} + \sqrt{a}$.

Solution: $\frac{\sqrt{3}}{3}$.
We have the following similarly ordered sequences:
$\sqrt{a}, \sqrt{b}, \sqrt{c}$
$\sqrt{ab}, \sqrt{ca}, \sqrt{bc}$

By the rearrangement inequality,

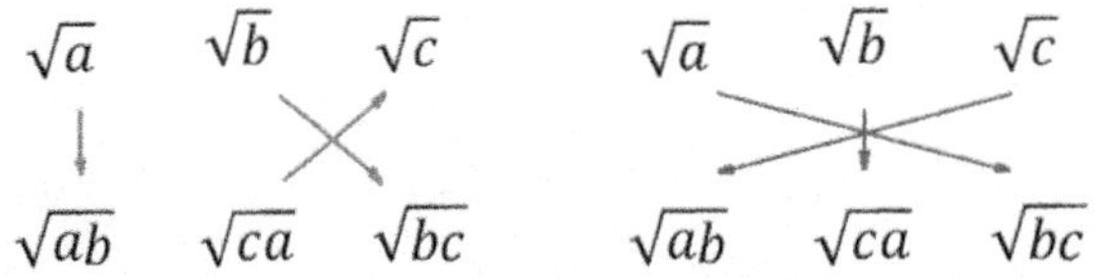

$$\begin{array}{ccc} \sqrt{a} & \sqrt{b} & \sqrt{c} \\ \downarrow & \times & \\ \sqrt{ab} & \sqrt{ca} & \sqrt{bc} \end{array} \qquad \begin{array}{ccc} \sqrt{a} & \sqrt{b} & \sqrt{c} \\ \sqrt{ab} & \sqrt{ca} & \sqrt{bc} \end{array}$$

$\sqrt{a} \cdot \sqrt{ab} + \sqrt{b} \cdot \sqrt{bc} + \sqrt{c} \cdot \sqrt{ca} \le \sqrt{a} \cdot \sqrt{bc} + \sqrt{b} \cdot \sqrt{ca} + \sqrt{c} \cdot \sqrt{ab}$

$\Rightarrow a\sqrt{b} + b\sqrt{c} + c\sqrt{a} \le 3\sqrt{abc} \le 3\sqrt{\frac{1}{27}} = \sqrt{\frac{1}{3}} = \frac{\sqrt{3}}{3}.$

The greatest value $\frac{\sqrt{3}}{3}$ is achieved when $a = b = c = \frac{1}{3}$.

Example 3. If a, b, and c are positive numbers with $a + b + c = 1$, find the greatest value of $\sqrt{ab} + \sqrt{bc} + \sqrt{ca}$.

Solution: 1.

Method 1:

We have the following similarly ordered sequences:

$\sqrt{a}, \sqrt{b}, \sqrt{c}$

$\sqrt{a}, \sqrt{b}, \sqrt{c}$

By the rearrangement inequality,

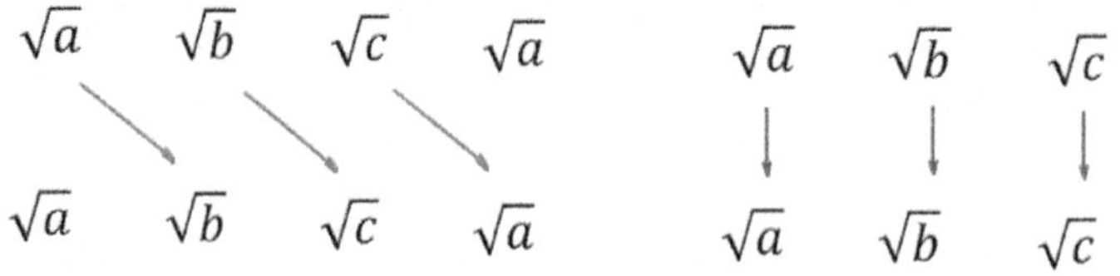

$$\begin{array}{cccc} \sqrt{a} & \sqrt{b} & \sqrt{c} & \sqrt{a} \\ \searrow & \searrow & \searrow & \\ \sqrt{a} & \sqrt{b} & \sqrt{c} & \sqrt{a} \end{array} \qquad \begin{array}{ccc} \sqrt{a} & \sqrt{b} & \sqrt{c} \\ \downarrow & \downarrow & \downarrow \\ \sqrt{a} & \sqrt{b} & \sqrt{c} \end{array}$$

$\sqrt{a} \cdot \sqrt{b} + \sqrt{b} \cdot \sqrt{c} + \sqrt{c} \cdot \sqrt{a} \le \sqrt{a} \cdot \sqrt{a} + \sqrt{b} \cdot \sqrt{b} + \sqrt{c} \cdot \sqrt{c}$, or

$\sqrt{ab} + \sqrt{bc} + \sqrt{ca} \le a + b + c = 1$

The greatest value 1 is achieved when $a = b = c = \frac{1}{3}$.

Method 2:

We know that

$2\sqrt{ab} \le a+b$ (1)

$2\sqrt{bc} \le b+c$ (2)

$2\sqrt{ca} \le c+a$ (3)

(1) + (2) + (3):

$2\sqrt{ab} + 2\sqrt{bc} + 2\sqrt{ac} \le (a+b)+(b+c)+(a+c) = 2$.

Therefore $\sqrt{ab} + \sqrt{bc} + \sqrt{ca} \le a + b + c = 1$

Example 4. Let a, b, $c \in R$ such that $a + b + c = 1$. Find the smallest value of $\frac{ab}{c} + \frac{bc}{a} + \frac{ca}{b}$.

Solution:

Since the inequality is symmetric, WLOG, we may assume that $a \le b \le c$.

Then we have the following two similarly ordered sequences:

ab, ac, bc

$\frac{1}{c}, \frac{1}{b}, \frac{1}{a}$.

By the rearrangement inequality, we have

ab	ca	bc		ab	ca	bc	ab
↓	↓	↓		↘	↘	↘	
$\frac{1}{c}$	$\frac{1}{b}$	$\frac{1}{a}$		$\frac{1}{c}$	$\frac{1}{b}$	$\frac{1}{a}$	$\frac{1}{c}$

$$\frac{ab}{c} + \frac{ca}{b} + \frac{bc}{a} \ge \frac{ab}{b} + \frac{ca}{a} + \frac{bc}{c} = a + b + c = 1.$$

The smallest value of 1 is achieved when $a = b = c = 1/3$.

Method 2:

$$\frac{ab}{c} + \frac{bc}{a} + \frac{ca}{b} = \frac{1}{2}\left(\frac{ab}{c} + \frac{bc}{a}\right) + \frac{1}{2}\left(\frac{bc}{a} + \frac{ca}{b}\right) + \frac{1}{2}\left(\frac{ca}{b} + \frac{ab}{c}\right).$$

By AM-GM, $\frac{1}{2}\left(\frac{ab}{c}+\frac{bc}{a}\right) \geq \sqrt{\frac{ab}{c}\cdot\frac{bc}{a}} = b.$

Similarly, we get:

$\frac{1}{2}\left(\frac{bc}{a}+\frac{ca}{b}\right) \geq \sqrt{\frac{bc}{a}\cdot\frac{ca}{b}} = c$, and $\frac{1}{2}\left(\frac{ca}{b}+\frac{ab}{c}\right) \geq \sqrt{\frac{ca}{b}\cdot\frac{ab}{c}} = a$

Adding them we get: $\frac{ab}{c}+\frac{bc}{a}+\frac{ca}{b} \geq a+b+c = 1.$

The smallest value of 1 is achieved when $a = b = c = 1/3$.

Example 5. Let $a, b, c \in R$ such that $a + b + c = 1$. Find the smallest value of

$\frac{a^2+b^2}{c}+\frac{b^2+c^2}{b}+\frac{c^2+a^2}{a}.$

Solution:

Since the inequality is symmetric, WLOG, we may assume that $a \leq b \leq c$.

Then we have the following two similarly ordered sequences:

$a^2+b^2, c^2+a^2, b^2+c^2$

$\frac{1}{c}, \frac{1}{b}, \frac{1}{a}.$

By the rearrangement inequality, we have

$$\begin{array}{ccc} a^2+b^2 & a^2+c^2 & b^2+c^2 \\ \downarrow & \downarrow & \downarrow \\ \frac{1}{c} & \frac{1}{b} & \frac{1}{a} \end{array} \qquad \begin{array}{cccc} a^2+b^2 & a^2+c^2 & b^2+c^2 & a^2+b^2 \\ \searrow & \searrow & \searrow & \\ \frac{1}{c} & \frac{1}{b} & \frac{1}{a} & \frac{1}{c} \end{array}$$

$$\frac{a^2+b^2}{c}+\frac{a^2+c^2}{b}+\frac{b^2+c^2}{a} \geq \frac{a^2+b^2}{b}+\frac{a^2+c^2}{a}+\frac{b^2+c^2}{c}$$
$$= \frac{a^2}{b}+\frac{c^2}{a}+\frac{b^2}{c}+a+b+c$$

We construct the following two similarly ordered sequences:

a^2, b^2, c^2

$\frac{1}{c}, \frac{1}{b}, \frac{1}{a}$.

By the rearrangement inequality, we have

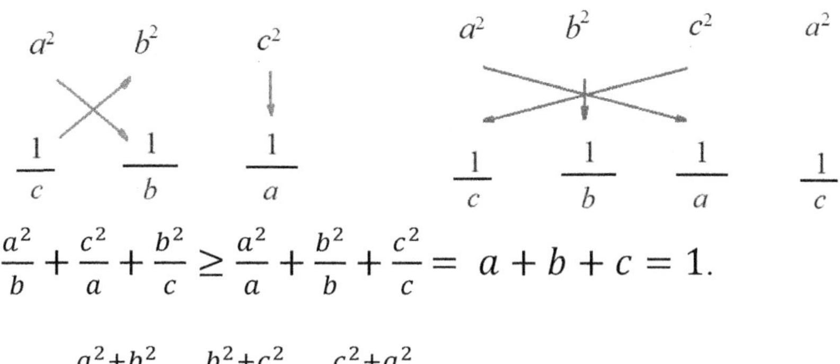

$$\frac{a^2}{b} + \frac{c^2}{a} + \frac{b^2}{c} \geq \frac{a^2}{a} + \frac{b^2}{b} + \frac{c^2}{c} = a + b + c = 1.$$

Thus $\frac{a^2+b^2}{c} + \frac{b^2+c^2}{b} + \frac{c^2+a^2}{a} \geq 2.$

The smallest value of 2 is achieved when $a = b = c = 1/3$.

Method 2:

$$\frac{a^2+b^2}{c} + \frac{b^2+c^2}{b} + \frac{c^2+a^2}{a} \geq 2\frac{ab}{c} + 2\frac{ca}{b} + 2\frac{bc}{a} = 2(\frac{ab}{c} + \frac{ca}{b} + \frac{bc}{a})$$

$$= 2[\frac{1}{2}\left(\frac{ab}{c} + \frac{bc}{a}\right) + \frac{1}{2}\left(\frac{ab}{c} + \frac{ca}{b}\right) + \frac{1}{2}\left(\frac{bc}{a} + \frac{ca}{b}\right)]$$

$$\geq 2\left(\sqrt{b^2} + \sqrt{a^2} + \sqrt{c^2}\right) = 2(a + b + c) = 2.$$

The smallest value of 2 is achieved when $a = b = c = 1/3$.

Example 6. (IMO long listed problems) Find the triples of positive integers x, y, and z satisfying $\frac{1}{x} + \frac{1}{y} + \frac{1}{z} = \frac{4}{5}$.

Solution: (2, 4, 20), and (2, 5, 10).

Since the equation is symmetric, WLOG, we let $x \le y \le z$ and we get

$$\frac{1}{x}+\frac{1}{x}+\frac{1}{x} \ge \frac{4}{5} > \frac{1}{x} \text{ or } \frac{3}{x} \ge \frac{4}{5} > \frac{1}{x}.$$

From this equation, we can determine the range for x: $2 \le x \le 3$.

Case I. $x = 2$. The original equation becomes $\frac{1}{2}+\frac{1}{y}+\frac{1}{z}=\frac{4}{5}$ or $\frac{1}{y}+\frac{1}{z}=\frac{4}{5}-\frac{1}{2}$ or

$$\frac{1}{y}+\frac{1}{z}=\frac{3}{10} \quad \Rightarrow \quad y=\frac{10z}{3z-10}.$$

$3z-10$ must be a factor of $10^2 = 2^2 \times 5^2$ or one of the factors: 1, 2, 4, 5, 10, 20, 25, 50, and 100.

Only $3z - 10 = 2$ and $3z - 10 = 5$ give integer values z, so we have the solutions (2, 4, 20) and (2, 5, 10).

Case II. $x = 3$. The original equation becomes $\frac{1}{y}+\frac{1}{z}=\frac{4}{5}-\frac{1}{3}$ or $\frac{1}{y}+\frac{1}{z}=\frac{7}{15}$

We get $y=\frac{15z}{7z-15}$, where $7z-15$ is a factor of $15^2 = 3^2 \times 5^2$, or one of the following factors: 1, 3, 5, 9, 15, 25, 45, 75, or 225.

We set $7z - 15$ to be the values of these factors, but after going through each factor, we see that z is not an integer for any of the factors.

So we have the solutions (2, 4, 20) and (2, 5, 10).

Example 7. Find all positive integer solutions to the equation: $x^x + y^y + z^z + u^u = w^w$.

Solution:

Since the equation is symmetric, WLOG, we let $x \le y \le z \le u$ and we get

$w \ge u + 1$ and $4u^u \ge w^w$, or $4 > 4 \cdot \frac{u^u}{(u+1)^u} \ge u + 1$

Thus $u < 3$. Since u is a positive integer, we have two cases:
(1) $u = 1$.
$x = y = z = 1, w = 2$.

(2) $u = 2$.
$x^x + y^y + z^z + 2^2 \le 4 \cdot 2^2 < 3^3 \le w^w$.
Therefore, the equation has only one set of solutions: $x = y = z = 1, w = 2$.

Example 8. Let a, b, c be positive real numbers such that $abc = 1$. Find the minimum value of $\frac{a^4+b^4}{a^3+b^3} + \frac{b^4+c^4}{b^3+c^3} + \frac{c^4+a^4}{c^3+a^3}$.

Solution:
By the rearrangement inequality
$a^n + b^n \ge a^{n-1}b + b^{n-1}a$ (1)

Adding $a^n + b^n$ to both sides of (1):
$2a^n + 2b^n \ge a^{n-1}b + b^{n-1}a + a^n + b^n$
Or $2a^n + 2b^n \ge (a^{n-1} + b^{n-1})(a + b) \quad \Rightarrow \quad \frac{a^n+b^n}{a^{n-1}+b^{n-1}} \ge \frac{a+b}{2}$.

Thus $\frac{a^4+b^4}{a^3+b^3} + \frac{b^4+c^4}{b^3+c^3} + \frac{c^4+a^4}{c^3+a^3} \ge \frac{a+b}{2} + \frac{b+c}{2} + \frac{c+a}{2} = a + b + c \ge 3\sqrt[3]{abc} = 3$.
The smallest value is 3 when $a = b = c = 1$.

CHAPTER 8. PROBLEMS

Problem 1. If $a, b, c \geq 0$, $a + b + c = 1$, find the greatest value of $(a+b)(b+c)(c+a)$.

Problem 2. If $a, b, c \geq 0$, $a^2 + b^2 + c^2 = 3$, find the greatest value of $a\sqrt{b} + b\sqrt{c} + c\sqrt{a}$.

Problem 3. If $a, b, c \geq 0$, $a + b + c = \sqrt{3}$, find the greatest value of $a\sqrt{bc} + b\sqrt{ca} + c\sqrt{ab}$.

Problem 4. Let $a, b, c \in \mathrm{R}$ such that $a^2 + b^2 + c^2 = 1$. Find the smallest value of $\frac{ab}{c} + \frac{bc}{a} + \frac{ca}{b}$.

Problem 5. If $a, b, c \geq 0$, find the smallest value of $\frac{a}{b+c} + \frac{b}{c+a} + \frac{c}{a+b}$.

Problem 6. Find the smallest positive value of $x + y + z$, where x, y, and z are different positive integers that satisfy this equation: $\frac{1}{x} + \frac{1}{y} + \frac{1}{z} = \frac{7}{10}$.

Problem 7. Find all positive integers w, x, y and z which satisfy $w! = x! + y! + z!$.

Problem 8. If $x_1, x_2, \ldots, x_n \geq 0$, $\sum_{i=1}^{n} x_i = 1$, find the smallest value of $\frac{{x_1}^2}{x_2} + \frac{{x_2}^2}{x_3} + {} + \cdots + \frac{{x_n}^2}{x_1}$.

CHAPTER 8. SOLUTIONS

Problem 1. Solution: $\frac{1}{3}$.

Method 1:

For the following similarly ordered sequences,

$a,\ \ b,\ \ c$

$a,\ \ b,\ \ c$

By the rearrangement inequality, we have

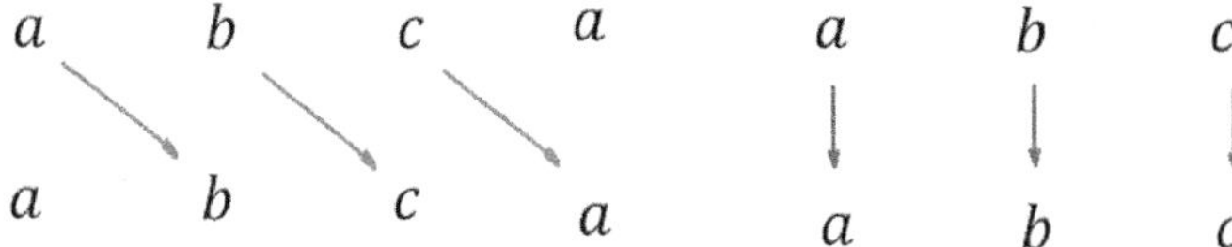

$(a+b)(b+c)(c+a) \le (a+a)(b+b)(c+c)$

$= 8abc \le 8 \cdot (\frac{a+b+c}{3})^3.$

$= \frac{8}{27}.$

The greatest value $\frac{8}{27}$ is achieved when $a = b = c = \frac{1}{3}$.

Method 2:

By AM-GM,

$(a+b)(b+c)(c+a) \le [\frac{2(a+b+c)}{3}]^3 = \frac{8}{27}.$

The greatest value $\frac{8}{27}$ is achieved when $a = b = c = \frac{1}{3}$.

Problem 2. Solution:

By Cauchy, $3 = a^2 + b^2 + c^2 \ge \frac{(a+b+c)^2}{3} \qquad \Rightarrow \qquad a + b + c \le 3.$

We have the following similarly ordered sequences:

$a, b, c.$

$\sqrt{a}, \sqrt{b}, \sqrt{c}$

By the rearrangement inequality,

$$\begin{matrix} a & b & c & a & & a & b & c \\ \searrow & \searrow & \searrow & & & \downarrow & \downarrow & \downarrow \\ \sqrt{a} & \sqrt{b} & \sqrt{c} & \sqrt{a} & & \sqrt{a} & \sqrt{b} & \sqrt{c} \end{matrix}$$

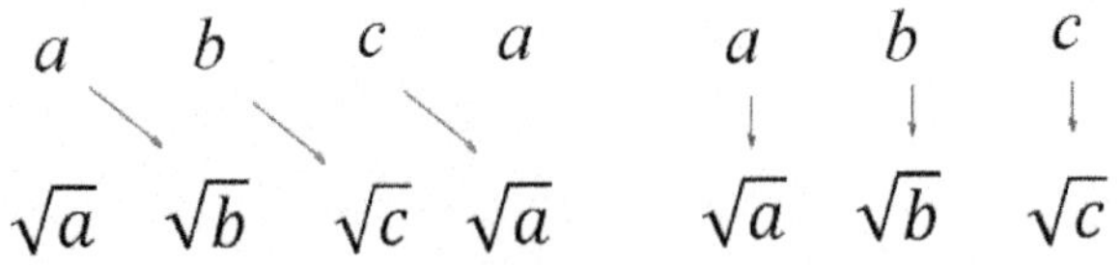

$a\sqrt{b} + b\sqrt{c} + c\sqrt{a} \le a\sqrt{a} + b\sqrt{b} + c\sqrt{c}$.

By Cauchy,

$a\sqrt{b} + b\sqrt{c} + c\sqrt{a} \le \sqrt{(a^2 + b^2 + c^2)(a + b + c)}$

$a\sqrt{a} + b\sqrt{b} + c\sqrt{c} \le \sqrt{(a^2 + b^2 + c^2)(a + b + c)}$

$(a\sqrt{b} + b\sqrt{c} + c\sqrt{a})(a\sqrt{a} + b\sqrt{b} + c\sqrt{c}) \le (a\sqrt{a} + b\sqrt{b} + c\sqrt{c})^2$
$\le (a^2 + b^2 + c^2)(a + b + c) \le 3 \cdot 3 = 9$.

Thus $a\sqrt{b} + b\sqrt{c} + c\sqrt{a} \le a\sqrt{a} + b\sqrt{b} + c\sqrt{c} \le 3$.

The greatest value is achieved when $a = b = c = 1$.

Problem 3. Solution:

Method 1:

We have the following similarly ordered sequences:

a, b, c.

$\sqrt{ab}, \sqrt{ac}, \sqrt{bc}$

By the rearrangement inequality,

$$\begin{matrix} a & b & c & & a & b & c \\ & \times & & & \downarrow & \times & \\ \sqrt{ab} & \sqrt{ca} & \sqrt{bc} & & \sqrt{ab} & \sqrt{ca} & \sqrt{bc} \end{matrix}$$

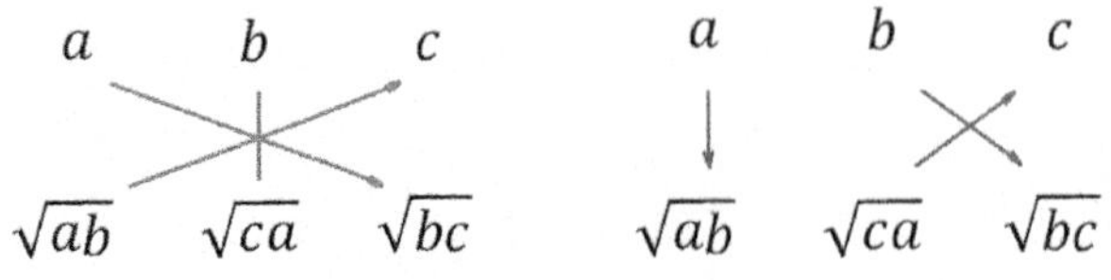

$a\sqrt{bc} + b\sqrt{ca} + c\sqrt{ab} \le a\sqrt{ab} + b\sqrt{bc} + c\sqrt{ca}$

$\le \sqrt{(a^2 + b^2 + c^2)(ab + bc + ca)}$

$\le \sqrt{(a + b + c)^2(ab + bc + ca)} \le \sqrt{3 \cdot \frac{1}{3}} = 1$.

The greatest value 1 is achieved when $a = b = c = \frac{\sqrt{3}}{3}$.

Method 2:

$$a\sqrt{bc} + b\sqrt{ca} + c\sqrt{ab} \le a \cdot \frac{b+c}{2} + b \cdot \frac{c+a}{2} + c \cdot \frac{a+b}{2} = ab + bc + ca$$

$\le \frac{(a+b+c)^2}{3} = \frac{3}{3} = 1.$

The greatest value is achieved when $a = b = c = \frac{\sqrt{3}}{3}$.

Problem 4. Solution: $\sqrt{3}$.

Since the inequality is symmetric, WLOG, we may assume that $a \le b \le c$.

Since $a \le b \le c$, we know that $ab \le ac \le bc$,

$\frac{ab}{c} \le \frac{ac}{b} \le \frac{bc}{a}$

Then we have the following two similarly ordered sequences:

$\frac{ab}{c}, \frac{ac}{b}, \frac{bc}{a}.$

$\frac{ab}{c}, \frac{ac}{b}, \frac{bc}{a}.$

By the rearrangement inequality, we have

$$\begin{array}{ccccccc} \frac{ab}{c} & \frac{ac}{b} & \frac{bc}{a} & \qquad \frac{ab}{c} & \frac{ac}{b} & \frac{bc}{a} & \frac{ab}{c} \\ \downarrow & \downarrow & \downarrow & \qquad \searrow & \searrow & \searrow & \\ \frac{ab}{c} & \frac{ac}{b} & \frac{bc}{a} & \qquad \frac{ab}{c} & \frac{ac}{b} & \frac{bc}{a} & \frac{ab}{c} \end{array}$$

$$(\frac{ab}{c})^2 + (\frac{ac}{b})^2 + (\frac{bc}{a})^2 \ge \frac{ab}{c} \cdot \frac{ac}{b} + \frac{ac}{b} \cdot \frac{bc}{a} + \frac{bc}{a} \cdot \frac{ab}{c} = a^2 + c^2 + b^2 = 1.$$

$$(\frac{ab}{c} + \frac{ca}{b} + \frac{bc}{a})^2 = (\frac{ab}{c})^2 + (\frac{ac}{b})^2 + (\frac{bc}{a})^2 + 2(\frac{ab}{c} \cdot \frac{ca}{b} + \frac{ac}{b} \cdot \frac{bc}{a} + \frac{bc}{a} \cdot \frac{ab}{c})$$

$\geq a^2 + c^2 + b^2 + 2(a^2 + c^2 + b^2) = 3.$

Thus $\frac{ab}{c} + \frac{bc}{a} + \frac{ca}{b} \geq \sqrt{3}.$

The smallest value of $\sqrt{3}$ is achieved when $a = b = c = \frac{\sqrt{3}}{3}$.

Method 2:

$$\left(\frac{ab}{c} + \frac{ca}{b} + \frac{bc}{a}\right)^2 = \frac{a^2b^2}{c^2} + \frac{b^2c^2}{a^2} + \frac{c^2a^2}{b^2} + 2(a^2 + b^2 + c^2)$$

$$= \frac{1}{2}\left(\frac{a^2b^2}{c^2} + \frac{c^2a^2}{b^2}\right) + \frac{1}{2}\left(\frac{b^2c^2}{a^2} + \frac{c^2a^2}{b^2}\right) + \frac{1}{2}\left(\frac{a^2b^2}{c^2} + \frac{b^2c^2}{a^2}\right) + 2$$

By AM-GM, $\frac{1}{2}\left(\frac{a^2b^2}{c^2} + \frac{c^2a^2}{b^2}\right) \geq \sqrt{\frac{a^2b^2}{c^2} \cdot \frac{c^2a^2}{b^2}} = a^2.$

Similarly, we get:

$\frac{1}{2}\left(\frac{b^2c^2}{a^2} + \frac{c^2a^2}{b^2}\right) \geq c^2$, and $\frac{1}{2}\left(\frac{a^2b^2}{c^2} + \frac{b^2c^2}{a^2}\right) \geq b^2$

Adding them we get: $\left(\frac{ab}{c} + \frac{ca}{b} + \frac{bc}{a}\right)^2 \geq a^2 + c^2 + b^2 + 2(a^2 + c^2 + b^2) = 3$

Thus $\frac{ab}{c} + \frac{bc}{a} + \frac{ca}{b} \geq \sqrt{3}.$

The smallest value of $\sqrt{3}$ is achieved when $a = b = c = \frac{\sqrt{3}}{3}$.

Problem 5. Solution:

Since the expression is a symmetric function of a, b, c, we can assume, without loss of generality, that $a \leq b \leq c$, and $\frac{1}{b+c} \leq \frac{1}{a+c} \leq \frac{1}{a+b}$.

$$\begin{array}{ccccccc} a & b & c & a & b & c & a \\ \downarrow & \downarrow & \downarrow & \searrow & \searrow & \searrow & \\ \frac{1}{b+c} & \frac{1}{c+a} & \frac{1}{a+b} & \frac{1}{b+c} & \frac{1}{c+a} & \frac{1}{a+b} & \frac{1}{b+c} \end{array}$$

$$\frac{a}{b+c} + \frac{b}{c+a} + \frac{c}{a+b} \geq \frac{c}{b+c} + \frac{a}{c+a} + \frac{b}{a+b} \qquad (1)$$

$a \quad b \quad c \qquad\qquad a \quad b \quad c \quad a$

$\downarrow \quad \downarrow \quad \downarrow \qquad\qquad \nearrow \quad \nearrow \quad \nearrow$

$\frac{1}{b+c} \quad \frac{1}{c+a} \quad \frac{1}{a+b} \qquad\qquad \frac{1}{b+c} \quad \frac{1}{c+a} \quad \frac{1}{a+b} \quad \frac{1}{b+c}$

$$\frac{a}{b+c}+\frac{b}{c+a}+\frac{c}{a+b} \geq \frac{b}{b+c}+\frac{c}{c+a}+\frac{a}{a+b} \qquad (2)$$

(1) + (2): $2\left(\frac{a}{b+c}+\frac{b}{c+a}+\frac{c}{a+b}\right) \geq \frac{b+c}{b+c}+\frac{c+a}{c+a}+\frac{a+b}{a+b}=3.$

Thus $\frac{a}{b+c}+\frac{b}{c+a}+\frac{c}{a+b} \geq \frac{3}{2}$

The smallest value is $\frac{3}{2}$ when $a=b=c=1$.

Problem 6. Solution: 14.

Since the equation is symmetric, WLOG, we let $x \leq y \leq z$ and we get

$$\frac{1}{x}+\frac{1}{x}+\frac{1}{x} \geq \frac{7}{10} > \frac{1}{x} \text{ or } \frac{3}{x} \geq \frac{7}{10} > \frac{1}{x}.$$

The range for x is: $\frac{30}{7} \geq x > \frac{10}{7}$.

So we have $2 \leq x \leq 4$.

Case I. If $x = 2$,

$$\frac{1}{2}+\frac{1}{y}+\frac{1}{z}=\frac{7}{10} \Rightarrow \frac{1}{y}+\frac{1}{z}=\frac{7}{10}-\frac{1}{2}=\frac{1}{5} \Rightarrow \frac{1}{y}+\frac{1}{z}=\frac{1}{5}$$

Since we only need to find out the smallest value of $x + y + z$, we only need to try to find values of y and z as close as possible.

Let $\frac{1}{y}+\frac{1}{z}=\frac{1}{5}=\frac{1}{10}+\frac{1}{10}$,

$x = 2$, $y = 10$, and $z = 10$.

Since x, y, and z must be different, we can rule out this case.

Case II. $x = 3$

$$\frac{1}{y}+\frac{1}{z}=\frac{7}{10}-\frac{1}{3}=\frac{11}{30}$$

$$\frac{1}{y}+\frac{1}{z}=\frac{11}{30}=\frac{5}{30}+\frac{6}{30}=\frac{1}{6}+\frac{1}{5},$$

$x = 3$, $y = 6$, and $z = 5$.

$x+y+z=14$

Case III. $x=4$

$$\frac{1}{y}+\frac{1}{z}=\frac{7}{10}-\frac{1}{4}=\frac{9}{20}=\frac{4}{20}+\frac{5}{20}=\frac{1}{5}+\frac{1}{4}$$

$x = 4$, $y = 5$, and $z = 4$

Since x, y, and z must be different, we can rule out this case. The least sum of x, y, and z is 14 from Case 2.

Problem 7. Solution:

Since the equation is symmetric, WLOG, we let $x \le y \le z$. Then $w \ge z+1$ so that $(z+1)z! = (z+1)! \le w! = x! + y! + z! \le 3z!$

Hence $z \le 2$.

A quick check shows that $x = y = z = 2$ and $w = 3$ form the only solution.

Problem 8. Solution:

method 1:

We have the following opposite ordered sequences:

$x_1{}^2, x_2{}^2, \cdots, x_{n-1}{}^2, x_n{}^2$

$\frac{1}{x_1}, \frac{1}{x_2}, \cdots, \frac{1}{x_{n-1}}, \frac{1}{x_n}$

By the rearrangement inequality,

$$\frac{x_1{}^2}{x_2}+\frac{x_2{}^2}{x_3}+\cdots+\frac{x_n{}^2}{x_1} \ge \frac{x_1{}^2}{x_1}+\frac{x_2{}^2}{x_2}+\cdots+\frac{x_n{}^2}{x_n} = x_1+x_2+\cdots+x_n = 1.$$

Method 2:

Since the expression is cyclic, we assume that one arrangement of $x_1, x_2, \ldots, x_n$ is $x_{i_1} \le x_{i_2} \le \cdots \le x_{i_{n-1}} \le x_{i_n}$, where $i_1, i_2, \ldots i_n$ is one of $1, 2, \ldots, n$.

Then we know that

$$x_{i_1}{}^2 \le x_{i_2}{}^2 \le \cdots \le x_{i_{n-1}}{}^2 \le x_{i_n}{}^2$$

$$\frac{1}{x_{i_1}} \ge \frac{1}{x_{i_2}} \ge \cdots \ge \frac{1}{x_{i_{n-1}}} \ge \frac{1}{x_{i_n}}$$

Thus we have the following opposite ordered sequences:

$$x_{i_1}{}^2, x_{i_2}{}^2, \cdots, x_{i_{n-1}}{}^2, x_{i_n}{}^2$$

$$\frac{1}{x_{i_1}}, \frac{1}{x_{i_2}}, \cdots, \frac{1}{x_{i_{n-1}}}, \frac{1}{x_{i_n}}$$

By the rearrangement inequality,

$$\frac{x_1{}^2}{x_2} + \frac{x_2{}^2}{x_3} + \cdots + \frac{x_n{}^2}{x_1} \ge \frac{x_{i_1}{}^2}{x_{i_1}} + \frac{x_{i_2}{}^2}{x_{i_2}} + \cdots + \frac{x_{i_{n-1}}{}^2}{x_{i_{n-1}}} + \frac{x_{i_n}{}^2}{x_{i_n}}$$

$$= x_{i_1} + x_{i_2} + \cdots + x_{i_{n-1}} + x_{i_n} = x_1 + x_2 + \cdots + x_n = 1.$$

Chapter 9 Proving Important Inequalities

We can easily prove many important inequalities such as AM-GM Inequality, Cauchy's Inequality, Chebyshev's inequality, and Schur's inequality. We will prove these inequalities in this section.

The *AM-GM* Inequality

(1) Two terms *AM-GM* Inequality

The arithmetic mean of two non-negative real numbers is greater than or equal to the geometric mean of the same list.

$\frac{a+b}{2} \ge \sqrt{ab}$ or $a+b \ge 2\sqrt{ab}$

Proof:

We have the following two similarly ordered sequences:

$\sqrt{a}$, $\sqrt{b}$

$\sqrt{a}$, $\sqrt{b}$

By the rearrangement inequality, we have

$$\begin{matrix} \sqrt{a} & \sqrt{b} \\ \downarrow & \downarrow \\ \sqrt{a} & \sqrt{b} \end{matrix} \qquad \begin{matrix} \sqrt{a} & & \sqrt{b} \\ & \times & \\ \sqrt{a} & & \sqrt{b} \end{matrix}$$

or $\begin{bmatrix} \sqrt{a} & \sqrt{b} \\ \sqrt{a} & \sqrt{b} \end{bmatrix} \ge \begin{bmatrix} \sqrt{a} & \sqrt{b} \\ \sqrt{b} & \sqrt{a} \end{bmatrix}$.

$$\sqrt{a}\cdot\sqrt{a}+\sqrt{b}\cdot\sqrt{b}=a+b\ge\sqrt{a}\cdot\sqrt{b}+\sqrt{a}\cdot\sqrt{b}=2\sqrt{ab},$$

where both a and b are nonnegative real numbers and equality occurs if and only if $a = b$.

(2) *n* terms *AM-GM* Inequality

In general, for n nonnegative real numbers $a_1, a_2, \ldots a_n$, we have the following AM-GM Inequality:

$$a_1 + a_2 + \ldots + a_n \ge n\sqrt[n]{a_1 \times a_2 \times \ldots \times a_n}$$

Equality occurs if and only if $a_1 = a_2 = \ldots = a_n$.

Proof:

Method 1:

We construct two opposite ordered sequences:

$$x_1 = \frac{a_1}{c},\ x_2 = \frac{a_1 a_2}{c^2},\ x_3 = \frac{a_1 a_2 a_3}{c^3}, \ldots,\ x_n = \frac{a_1 a_2 a_3 \cdots a_n}{c^n} = 1,$$

$$y_1 = \frac{1}{x_1},\ y = \frac{1}{x_2},\ y_3 = \frac{1}{x_3}, \ldots,\ y_n = \frac{1}{x_n} = 1.$$

Since x_i and y_i are reciprocal, thus

$x_1 y_1 + x_2 y_2 + \cdots + x_n y_n \le x_1 y_n + x_2 y_2 + \cdots + x_n y_{n-1}$,

that is $1 + 1 + \cdots + 1 \le \frac{a_1}{c} + \frac{a_2}{c} + \ldots + \frac{a_n}{c} \quad \Rightarrow$

$n \le \frac{a_1}{c} + \frac{a_2}{c} + \ldots + \frac{a_n}{c} = \frac{a_1 + a_2 + \cdots + a_n}{c}$, or $c \le \frac{a_1 + a_2 + \cdots + a_n}{n}$, that is

$$a_1 + a_2 + \ldots + a_n \ge n\sqrt[n]{a_1 \times a_2 \times \ldots \times a_n}$$

The equality holds when $x_1 = x_2 = \cdots x_n$, or $a_1 = a_2 = \cdots a_n$.

WLOG, we assume that $a_1 a_2 a_3 \cdots a_n = 1$.

Let $a_1 = \frac{x_1}{x_2},\ a_2 = \frac{x_2}{x_3},\ \ldots,\ a_{n-1} = \frac{x_{n-1}}{x_n},\ x_1, x_2, \ldots x_n > 0$, then $a_n = \frac{x_n}{x_1}$.

The problem becomes

$$\frac{x_1}{x_2} + \frac{x_2}{x_3} + \ldots + \frac{x_{n-1}}{x_n} + \frac{x_n}{x_1} \ge n.$$

Note that if the sequence $(x_1, x_2, \ldots x_n)$ is increasing, then the sequence $(\frac{1}{x_1}, \frac{1}{x_2}, \ldots, \frac{1}{x_n})$ will be decreasing.

By the rearrangement inequality, we have

$$\frac{x_1}{x_2}+\frac{x_2}{x_3}+\ldots+\frac{x_{n-1}}{x_n}+\frac{x_n}{x_1}\geq\frac{x_1}{x_1}+\frac{x_2}{x_2}+\ldots+\frac{x_n}{x_n}=1+1+1+\cdots+1=n.$$

Chebyshev's inequality

(a) If the sequences $(a_1, a_2, \ldots, a_n)$ and $(b_1, b_2, \ldots, b_n)$ are similarly ordered, then

$$\frac{a_1b_1+a_2b_2+\cdots+a_nb_n}{n}\geq\frac{a_1+a_2+a_3+\cdots+a_n}{n}\cdot\frac{b_1+b_2+b+\cdots+b_n}{n}$$

(b) If the sequences $(a_1, a_2, \ldots, a_n)$ and $(b_1, b_2, \ldots, b_n)$ are oppositely ordered, then

$$\frac{a_1b_1+a_2b_2+\cdots+a_nb_n}{n}\leq\frac{a_1+a_2+a_3+\cdots+a_n}{n}\cdot\frac{b_1+b_2+b+\cdots+b_n}{n}$$

Proof:

We prove (a):

$$\frac{a_1b_1+a_2b_2+\cdots+a_nb_n}{n}\geq\frac{a_1+a_2+a_3+\cdots+a_n}{n}\cdot\frac{b_1+b_2+b+\cdots+b_n}{n}$$

Since the sequences are similarly ordered, $a_1 \leq a_2 \leq \ldots \leq a_n$; $b_1 \leq b_2 \leq \ldots \leq b_n$, by the rearrangement inequality, we have

$a_1b_1 + a_2 b_2 + \ldots a_nb_n \geq a_1b_1 + a_2 b_2 + \ldots + a_nb_n$
$a_1b_1 + a_2 b_2 + \ldots a_nb_n \geq a_1b_2 + a_2 b_2 + \ldots + a_nb_1$
$a_1b_1 + a_2 b_2 + \ldots a_nb_n \geq a_1b_3 + a_2 b_4 + \ldots + a_nb_2$
....

$a_1b_1 + a_2 b_2 + \ldots a_nb_n \geq a_1b_n + a_2 b_1 + \ldots a_nb_{n-1}$

Adding the above inequalities we get:
$n(a_1b_1 + a_2 b_2 + \ldots a_nb_n) \geq (a_1 + a_2 + \ldots + a_n)(b_1 + b_2 + \ldots + b_n)$

Dividing the above inequality by n^2:

$$\frac{a_1b_1+a_2b_2+\cdots+a_nb_n}{n} \geq \frac{a_1+a_2+a_3+\cdots+a_n}{n} \cdot \frac{b_1+b_2+b+\cdots+b_n}{n}.$$

Similarly we can prove (b).

Cauchy's Inequality

Let $a_1, a_2, \ldots, a_n,$ and $b_1, b_2, \ldots, b_n$ be real numbers. Then
$(a_1b_1 + a_2b_2 + \cdots + a_nb_n)^2 \leq ({a_1}^2 + {a_2}^2 + \cdots + {a_n}^2)({b_1}^2 + {b_2}^2 + \cdots + {b_n}^2)$

Equality occurs if and only if $b_i = 0\,(i = 1, 2, \ldots, n)$ or $a_i = kb_i(i = 1, 2, \ldots, n)$.

Proof:
Let the sequences $(a_1, a_2, \ldots, a_n)$ and $(b_1, b_2, \ldots, b_n)$ are oppositely ordered, then by the rearrangement inequality, we have

$$\frac{a_1b_1+a_2b_2+\cdots+a_nb_n}{n} \leq \frac{a_1+a_2+\cdots+a_n}{n} \cdot \frac{b_1+b_2+\cdots+b_n}{n}$$

We know by AM-GM that

$$a_1+a_2+\cdots+a_n = \sqrt{(a_1+a_2+\cdots+a_n)^2} \leq \sqrt{n({a_1}^2 + {a_2}^2 + \cdots + {a_n}^2)}$$

$$b_1+b_2+\cdots+b_n = \sqrt{(b_1+b_2+\cdots+b_n)^2} \leq \sqrt{n({b_1}^2 + {b_2}^2 + \cdots + {b_n}^2)}$$

Thus $\frac{a_1+a_2+a_3+\cdots+a_n}{n} \cdot \frac{b_1+b_2+b+\cdots+b_n}{n} \leq \frac{\sqrt{n({a_1}^2+{a_2}^2+\cdots+{a_n}^2)}}{n} \cdot \frac{\sqrt{n({b_1}^2+{b_2}^2+\cdots+{b_n}^2)}}{n}$

$$= \frac{\sqrt{n({a_1}^2 + {a_2}^2 + \cdots + {a_n}^2) \cdot n({b_1}^2 + {b_2}^2 + \cdots + {b_n}^2)}}{n^2}$$

$$= \frac{\sqrt{({a_1}^2+{a_2}^2+\cdots+{a_n}^2)\cdot({b_1}^2+{b_2}^2+\cdots+{b_n}^2)}}{n}.$$

Then we can have

$$\frac{a_1b_1+a_2b_2+\cdots+a_nb_n}{n} \leq \frac{\sqrt{({a_1}^2+{a_2}^2+\cdots+{a_n}^2)\cdot({b_1}^2+{b_2}^2+\cdots+{b_n}^2)}}{n}$$

Squaring both sides of the above inequality, we get:
$(a_1b_1 + a_2b_2 + \cdots + a_nb_n)^2 \le ({a_1}^2 + {a_2}^2 + \cdots + {a_n}^2)({b_1}^2 + {b_2}^2 + \cdots + {b_n}^2)$

Schur's inequality

Let a, b, c be nonnegative numbers with $r \ge 0$. Then
$a^r(a-b)(a-c) + b^r(b-c)(b-a) + c^r(c-a)(c-b) \ge 0.$

Proof:
Schur's inequality is the general examples of "the arrange in order" principle
So we can deduce Schur's inequality from the rearrangement inequality.

Since the inequality is symmetric in a, b, c, we may assume without loss of generality that $a \le b \le c$. Then the inequality
$a^r(a-b)(a-c) + (c-b)[c^r(c-a) - b^r(b-a)] \ge 0.$
clearly holds, since every term on the left-hand side of the inequality is non-negative. This rearranges to Schur's inequality.
Equality holds if and only if $a = b = c$ or some two of a, b, c are equal and the other is 0.

References

1. Arthur Engel, Problem-Solving Strategies 1998 Springer-Verlag New York

2. R. B. Manfrino, J. A. G. Ortega and R. V. Delgado, Inequalities A Mathematical Olympiad Approach 2009 Birkhäuser Verlag AG

3. Samin Riasat, Basics of Olympiad Inequalities. 2008

5. Pham Kim Hung, Secrets in Inequalities (volume 1) GIL Publishing House 2007.

4. Z. Cvetkovski, Inequalities: Theorems, Techniques and Selected Problems, Springer-Verlag Berlin Heidelberg 2012

6. G. Hardy, J. E. Littlewood and G. Polya, Inequalities, Cambridge University Press, Cambridge, 1934.

7. Holden Lee Rearrangement Inequality 2011.

8. 张宁生，田利英 绝对不等式 200 例 新华出版社 1990.

9. Thomas J. Mildorf Olympiad Inequalities 2005.

10. Dragos Hrimiuc The Rearrangement Inequality 2000.

11. Evan Chen A Brief Introduction to Olympiad Inequalities 2014.

12. 南山 柯西不等式与排序不等式 上海教育出版社 1996.

13. Law Ka Ho Variation and generalizations to the rearrangement inequality Mathematical Excalibur, January 2015.

Index

Printed in Great Britain
by Amazon